Childhood Neurologic Problems

Childhood Neurologic Problems
A Textbook for Health Care Professionals

Doris A. Trauner, M.D.
Assistant Professor of Neurology and Pediatrics
Director, Learning Evaluation Clinic
University of California Medical Center
San Diego, California

Year Book Medical Publishers, Inc.
CHICAGO • LONDON

Copyright © 1979 by Year Book Medical Publishers, Inc. All rights reserved. No part of this publication may be reproduced, stored in a retrieval system, or transmitted, in any form or by any means, electronic, mechanical, photocopying, recording, or otherwise, without prior written permission from the publisher. Printed in the United States of America.

Library of Congress Cataloging in Publication Data

Trauner, Doris A
    Childhood neurologic problems.

    Includes index.
    1. Pediatric neurology.   I. Title.   [DNLM:
1. Nervous system diseases — In infancy and childhood.
WS340.3 T777c]
RJ486.T73   618.9'28   79-12868
ISBN 0-8151-8832-3

To my husband Dick —
for everything

FOREWORD

An understanding of pediatric neurology is essential to the understanding and management of a large number of children with a variety of problems. This follows from the central position of the nervous system in directing other functions and its vulnerability to the effects of disease, injury or toxin. All of us who take care of children need to know a certain amount of pediatric neurology. I have long been interested in having a concise source of information that covered the breadth of the field. Doctor Trauner has provided us with just this. This book was written with a broad audience of health care professionals in mind—nurses, physiotherapists, speech pathologists, anyone who deals with children with problems involving the nervous system. I believe that the book will also be useful to physicians in family practice and pediatrics.

Dr. Doris Trauner is a dedicated physician, concerned daily with the problems of children with neurologic disorders. She has done original work in pediatric neurology from the time she was a medical student at the Medical College of Virginia. Doctor Trauner is now Assistant Professor of Neurology and Pediatrics at the University of California San Diego and is one of the world's authorities on Reye's syndrome.

Among her many talents is Dr. Trauner's real skill as a teacher. She is good at making complicated things understandable to students and to the rest of us. I feel that in this book she has selected the important issues in pediatric neurology and that she has presented them with the clarity that will make this book useful to a broad audience of health care professionals.

WILLIAM L. NYHAN, M.D., PH.D.
Professor and Chairman, Department of Pediatrics
University of California, San Diego

PREFACE

MANY PROFESSIONALS are involved in the care, education and rehabilitation of children with neurologic disorders. Physical, occupational and speech therapists, school nurses, teachers and educational psychologists—all must deal with the special problems that such children present. Understanding of neurologic dysfunction and its implications for the child's future life sometimes is incomplete. Many of the afflictions of the nervous system are rare and may be new to the person called on to deal with the results. Often, medications have been prescribed that may alter the child's educational or therapeutic response. A reference source that deals with these problems would be a useful guide to all those involved in the care of such a child.

During the time that I spent as a pediatric neurology consultant at the Brandecker-Ridge Easter Seals Treatment Center in Chicago, Illinois, I became aware of a problem. Personnel at the Center were dedicated and well trained and desired to know more about their patients' diagnoses in order to treat them most effectively. But we could find no single text that discussed neurologic disorders, treatment and outcome in a concise, readable and thorough manner. This book was undertaken partly through the impetus of these dedicated people.

The purpose of this text is to provide professionals involved in the care of the neurologically disabled child with a comprehensive guide to childhood neurologic problems; what they mean to the patient, family and professional; and a discussion of treatments used for the more commonly encountered disorders. It is hoped that with the expertise of the professionals who read this book, such children will have a brighter future.

Numerous people have been involved in the preparation of

this book, either directly or indirectly. Dr. William Nyhan, Chairman of the Department of Pediatrics at the University of California, San Diego, has been a continuing source of wisdom, guidance and enthusiasm ever since my internship in his department. Dr. Peter Huttenlocher, my mentor in pediatric neurology, shared willingly his tremendous knowledge of this field. His dynamic teaching and love for pediatric neurology have attracted many of his students into this specialty.

My good friends and professional associates in the Communicative Disorders Center at UCSD, with Mrs. Carol Grote as Director, have taught me much about rehabilitation of children with neurologic handicaps. The importance of their work is too often underestimated, but the children they treat are well aware of the benefits of rehabilitative therapy.

Ms. Valerie Lockhart spent many long hours in manuscript preparation, managing to do an excellent job despite constant interruptions. Mrs. Beverly Gonsowski donated her time to this effort as well.

I want to thank Drs. William Nyhan, Hector James, Marjorie Seybold, Ray Skoglund and James Connor, Mrs. Carol Grote and Susan Lingle for reviewing certain chapters and for their constructive criticisms. A very special note of thanks goes to Dr. Paul Schultz for his thorough and constructive review of the entire manuscript.

All the drawings in the text were done by Ms. Penelope Roberts.

DORIS A. TRAUNER, M.D.

CONTENTS

1. Normal Neurologic Development 1
2. The Neurologic Examination 12
3. Seizure Disorders 21
4. Headaches in Children 33
5. Structural Diseases of the Nervous System . . 42
6. Mental Retardation 58
7. Genetic and Metabolic Disorders 69
8. Degenerative Diseases of the
   Nervous System 85
9. Cerebral Palsy 90
10. Nerve and Muscle Diseases 103
11. Infections of the Central Nervous System . . 116
12. Hyperactivity Syndromes 125
13. Learning Disabilities 133
14. Speech and Language Disorders 141

    Index 153

1

NORMAL NEUROLOGIC DEVELOPMENT

ANY UNDERSTANDING of the child with neurologic problems must begin with some knowledge of normal neurologic development. This chapter will offer a brief discussion of brain anatomy. With that background, we then will turn to normal development from birth to early school years.

The brain is a complex structure, both anatomically and functionally. Anatomic examination of a brain reveals that it is divided into several parts (Fig. 1–1). The earliest area to develop is the brainstem, which is located at the base of the brain. This structure contains fiber tracts connecting other parts of the brain with the spinal cord; groups of cells called cranial nerve nuclei, which are responsible for such functions as smell, movement of eye and facial muscles, pupillary responses and hearing; and vital centers for control of heart rate and respiration.

The spinal cord projects downward from the brainstem and is encased in a bony covering, the vertebral column or spine. The spinal cord sends out projections from nerve cells to muscles and joints, and carries nerve fibers which control bowel and bladder function as well as sensation and strength, under control from cells inside the brain.

Immediately adjacent to and partially covering the brainstem is the cerebellum, which is a center for muscle tone and coordination.

The cortex is located above the brainstem, and in humans makes up the largest part of the brain. It is divided into right and left cerebral hemispheres and contains many folds. Each indentation on the surface is called a *sulcus*, and the section of cortex between two sulci is called a *gyrus*.

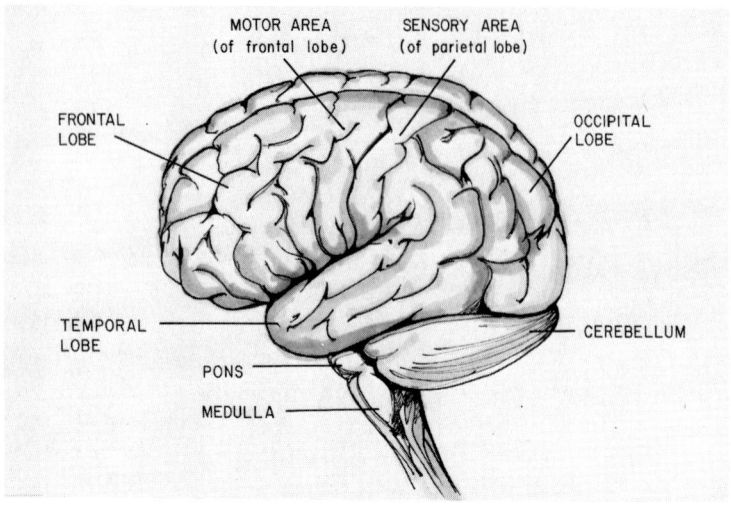

Fig. 1-1.—Diagrammatic representation of the brain and its major divisions in lateral view.

The cortex is further divided into lobes: frontal, parietal, temporal and occipital. Each lobe has certain primary functions to carry out, e.g., the frontal lobe is responsible for motor control.

In the interior of the brain there is a connecting system of fluid-filled spaces called *ventricles*. These contain cerebrospinal fluid, which bathes the brain.

The entire brain is surrounded by a thin layer of fluid and then by several thin coverings called *meninges*. Blood vessels course throughout the brain itself as well as over the surface, carrying necessary nutrients to brain cells.

The brain is encased in a bony covering—the *cranium*, or skull. The cranium is made up of several bones that are separate from one another at birth but which fuse over the first few years of life to form a solid bone.

The points at which two cranial bones meet are called *sutures*. In the infant there are two roughly diamond-shaped gaps between the bones called the *anterior* and *posterior fontanelles*. The posterior fontanelle closes soon after birth but the anterior fontanelle ("soft spot" on top of the head) remains open until 12–18 months of age.

The major part of brain growth occurs in the first year of life. By the end of the first year, the brain is approximately two-thirds of adult size and by the end of the second year is about four-fifths that of the adult brain.

Any abnormality (such as infection, biochemical imbalance, trauma) that upsets the brain's development and growth during this period can exert profound effects on eventual brain function. Therefore, early neurologic evaluation of potential difficulties is important in assessing the nature and extent of any problem and in instituting treatment, when available, to prevent further damage to the growing brain.

Head size reflects brain size; if the brain is damaged and stops growing, the bones have no stimulus to grow and the individual bones of the skull will fuse prematurely, causing a small head, or *microcephaly*. Conversely, if there is increased pressure in the brain, as from an obstruction to fluid reabsorption or an increase in production of fluid, the head will grow more rapidly than normal and produce hydrocephalus. The normal head circumference for the full-term newborn infant is 35 centimeters (13¾ inches).

BIRTH TO 6 MONTHS

In the newborn, higher cortical function has not yet developed and most of the neurologic examination is directed toward assessment of the more primitive parts of the nervous system. The normal newborn can perform most basic functions, but at times to a limited degree. For example, the newborn infant blinks at bright lights, and pupils will constrict if a bright light is held near the eyes. The infant will also turn toward a light and blink at a loud sound.

The newborn infant is able to yawn, sneeze, cough and hiccup. All of these reflex functions require an intact brainstem. The infant responds to pain by withdrawal of the stimulated area and issues a cry of discomfort. In a prone position he can lift his head slightly and turn it from side to side.

Certain reflexes are present in the normal newborn infant

that disappear as the brain matures. These reflexes are conducted through the more primitive parts of the brain and are inhibited as the more advanced cortical functions and voluntary control take over. Persistence of these immature reflexes after the normal age of disappearance of each reflex indicates some cortical dysfunction. Three of these reflexes are described here along with the method used to elicit them.

TONIC NECK REFLEX (Fig. 1–2).—With the infant lying on his back, the examiner turns the head briskly to one side. On the side to which the face is turned, the arm and leg extend, while the limbs on the opposite side flex at the same time. This reflex usually is incomplete in the mature newborn and disappears at about the fourth month of life. It is necessary to be able to overcome this reflex before the infant can roll over and sit up. An asymmetry in the reflex or persistence past 4–6 months of age, or a complete reflex in a mature infant, suggests a cerebral abnormality.

MORO REFLEX (Fig. 1–3).—This reflex is induced by making a loud noise near the infant or by supporting the back and dropping the head slightly. It is characterized by generalized extension of all four limbs followed by flexion of the limbs. The fingers fan out and the infant cries. This reflex usually is present in the full-term newborn and gradually disappears over the first 4–6 months of life.

Fig. 1–2.—Tonic neck reflex in a normal infant.

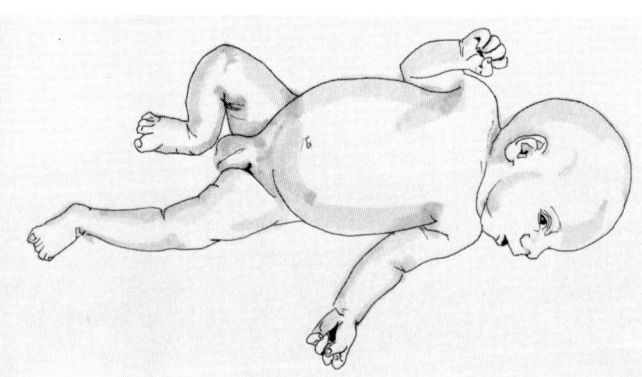

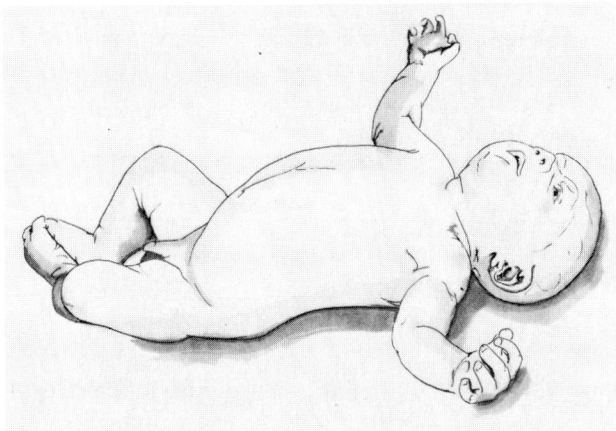

Fig. 1–3.—Moro reflex.

PLACING AND STEPPING REFLEXES.—If the infant is held upright and the feet are allowed to touch the table, a newborn infant will have automatic stepping reflexes. If the infant is lifted suddenly and the feet again are placed on the table, the baby will have an extensor thrust of the legs to support him-

TABLE 1–1.—ACQUISITION OF SKILLS DURING FIRST YEAR OF LIFE

Newborn	Fixes on light
	Grasp reflex
	Moro reflex
3 months	Social smile
	Good head control
6 months	Rolls over
	Reaches for and transfers object
	Sits with minimal support
	Laughs out loud
9 months	Pincer grasp
	Sits alone
	Stands with support
	Crawls
	Makes repetitive sounds ("da-da")
12 months	Walks with minimal support
	Crawls
	Uses 3–4 words
	Imitates behavior (waves "bye-bye")
	Plays peekaboo

self. These reflexes disappear as the child begins voluntary walking during the first year of life.

The acquisition and disappearance of these reflexes and other developmental milestones now will be discussed in chronologic order (Table 1-1).

DEVELOPMENTAL MILESTONES FROM BIRTH TO 6 MONTHS OF LIFE

If the newborn infant is placed face down (prone) on the table or bed he is able to turn his head from side to side. By 4 weeks of age he can lift his head above the surface of the bed. The newborn is also able to fix on a light or a bright object in the first days of life and is able to follow it with his eyes for a few degrees. By the end of the second month he can follow the light all the way to the right or left. In the first 4-8 weeks of life, if the infant is pulled from lying to sitting, the head lags (Fig. 1-4); in the upright position, head control is poor. By 12 weeks of age there is some head control while being pulled to sitting, but the head may not be fully upright when the infant is placed in the sitting position.

A normal infant displays a grasp reflex; that is, if an object is placed in the palm of his hand, he will automatically grasp it. This reflex persists until about 8 weeks of age, after which voluntary grasp begins to take over. By 12 weeks of age, the child should attempt to grasp an object that is held near him and may hold it briefly if contact is made with the hand.

By 8 weeks of age, most infants have a social smile; by 3 months, the child makes some noises indicating pleasure on social contact. A social smile should be present by 12 weeks of age.

By 3 months of age, the child who is lying face down can lift his head and chest off the surface of the bed with his arms extended in front of him. By 4 months of age he is able to raise his head to an upright position and turn it from side to side. Between 3 and 4 months, the infant begins to bring his hands to the midline or to the mouth. At this time, the child also begins to make contact with objects brought within his reach and may bring these to the midline or to his mouth to explore

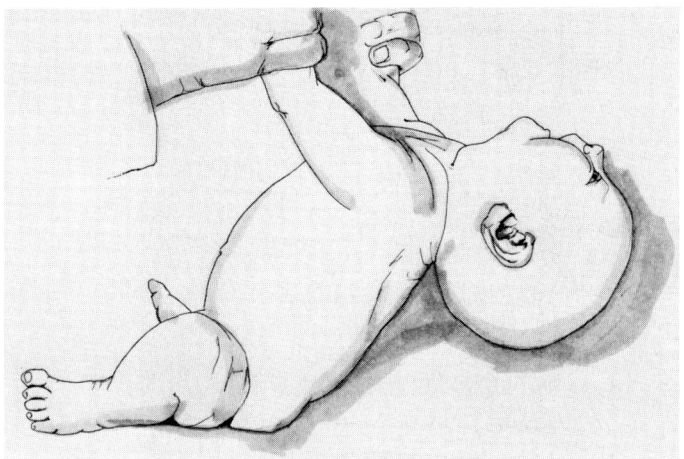

Fig. 1–4. – Normal head lag in a 2-week-old infant.

them. There no longer is any head lag when the child is brought to a sitting position, and the head is held steady and upright without bobbing when the child is standing or sitting. The infant also begins to enjoy being supported upright and is much more attracted to objects in his environment. He is beginning to be able to look around and to grasp an object of moderate size, such as a rattle or a ball.

By 5–6 months, the child has begun to roll over, first from front to back and then in the reverse position. By 6 months he often is able to sit alone, leaning forward on his hands or with only slight support at his back. At this age he can also use his thumb to oppose his fingers and can grasp an object and transfer it from one hand to the other. He now can be pulled from a sitting to a standing position and will support his weight on his extended legs.

A child of this age is much more responsive to social contact and he will laugh out loud when given attention or he may show signs of displeasure if pleasant contact is terminated. He begins to show preference for the person giving him most of his care.

At the end of 6 months, the normal infant no longer has tonic neck reflexes or a Moro reflex and no longer has a reflex grasp.

The child now can roll over and sit, at least with support, has good head control and reaches for and transfers objects from hand to hand. He is social and laughs out loud and at times makes cooing noises.

6–12 MONTHS

By this time, the normal infant is much more interested in his immediate environment and in his own body. The child will begin to show interest in his legs and feet and will play with them when lying on his back. Between 6 and 9 months, the hand movements become much more coordinated in that the infant can use his thumb and forefinger in a pincer grasp to get smaller objects. By 8–9 months he can sit up without assistance and by 9–10 months is beginning to creep and crawl. At this age he may be able to stand for a few seconds if the hands alone are supported and by 9 months he can take a few steps with the hands held.

Speech development progresses rapidly at this age also. The infant of 8 months makes repetitive sounds such as ma-ma and da-da. At this age he recognizes his own name and by 1 year of age he can show by his behavior that he knows the names of some objects. By 1 year of age he may meaningfully use 1–4 words other than ma-ma and da-da.

During the second 6 months of life, the infant shows some degree of social differentiation, preferring his mother and reacting negatively to strangers. There is some degree of dependence on his mother, although as the infant becomes more mobile there is less dependence on her physical presence. At this age, the child also becomes aware that an object that is covered up still is there, and peekaboo becomes an enjoyable game.

Imitative behavior begins during this time. The child may begin to imitate waving bye-bye and throwing a ball.

By 1 year of age, the infant has made considerable progress in gaining independence. He can walk or at least crawl, use a few words, laugh and play. The nervous system has matured tremendously and the child is ready to acquire the more sophisticated motor skills of the second year.

SECOND YEAR OF LIFE

During the second year of life, the child changes rapidly. By 15 months he is able to walk alone and by 18 months he can run stiffly. At 18 months he can climb steps with one hand held and one step at a time; that is, he does not yet alternate feet. By 20 months he can go down steps. By 24 months, the child can run well without falling.

Fine motor skills, including eye-hand coordination, improve rapidly as well. By 12 months of age, the infant can reach for a small object and then release it into the hand of a person requesting it. By 15 months he can put one cube on top of another after being shown; by 18 months he can make a 3-cube tower and by 24 months a 6-cube tower. At 18 months he can scribble and imitate vertical lines.

Speech progresses at a more variable rate than other motor skills. Many children will not make intelligible words until 18 months of age. These children often have a large amount of baby talk that is unintelligible to others. By 18 months of age, however, they should have approximately 10 words of intelligible speech and by 24 months should be able to make a 3-word sentence.

Toilet training usually can be undertaken during the latter part of the second year, since such needs now can be verbalized.

By the end of 2 years, the normal child can run, kick a ball, speak 2- to 3-word sentences and is toilet trained. He has gained relative motor and social independence.

THIRD TO FIFTH YEAR

During this time, further refinement of motor skills takes place. Between the second and third year, the child learns to coordinate feet and hands more skillfully and by 3 years of age can alternate feet to climb stairs. He can stand for a short time on one foot. Most children can ride a tricycle by 3–4 years of age. By 3 years, the child enjoys scribbling with a pencil or crayons, and can copy a drawing of a circle or a cross after being shown how to do it (Table 1–2).

TABLE 1-2.—AGE AT WHICH DESIGN COPYING SKILLS ARE ACHIEVED

DESIGN	AGE IN YEARS
○	3
+	3½-4
□	4½-5
△	5-5½
◇	6-7

Speech development progresses rapidly also. By 3 years, most of the consonants have been mastered and are about 75% intelligible. By 4 years of age, speech should be intelligible almost all the time and the child is able to use some adjectives and adverbs. Speech is relatively intact by the age of 5.

The 4-year-old is able to draw a cross and a circle without a demonstration. He can count 4 objects and is able to alternate feet descending stairs. He is able to jump or hop with both feet together. By the time the child is of school age he is able to run, hop and is beginning to learn to skip; he can draw a square and a triangle. He uses speech fluently. Recognition of colors, which may come about as early as the third year, definitely should be present by the fifth year of age.

EARLY SCHOOL YEARS

Between the ages of 6 and 12, the child is engaged in vigorous physical and mental activity. Motor skills become more directed toward organized activities such as writing, drawing and sports. Since the child spends a large portion of his time away from home, he begins to function more independently of his parents. Skills such as reading, writing, spelling and arithmetic are learned during this time and present no problem to the normal child. Speech is well structured in this age period and abstract concepts now can be understood by the child. It is also at this time that neurologic deficits become most obvious, since many people are concentrating on teaching the child. The child with a learning disability or other neurologic handicap should be treated in such a way that the tasks he *can* accomplish are emphasized, while at the same time concentration is focused on areas that will present special problems. In this way, the child's potential can be maximized.

Once normal neurologic development is understood, we can go on to recognizing aberrations from this norm. This is the subject of the following chapters.

2

THE NEUROLOGIC EXAMINATION

A CHILD is referred to a pediatric neurologist for many reasons. The most common problems include poor school performance, behavior problems, poor motor skills (for example, "clumsiness"), headaches, convulsions, lethargy or inattentiveness. The neurologist relies on descriptions of behavior from parents, teachers and school nurses. He then takes the complete history from the parent. Areas of questioning include specific developmental milestones: for example, at what age did the child roll over, sit, walk and talk? Has there been a change in the child's rate of development; that is, did he progress normally up to a certain age and then slow down? Did he lose abilities once acquired? Or was he always slow to do things? The answers to these questions can help to differentiate psychomotor delay or retardation from acquired and possibly progressive or degenerative diseases. A child who has been slow from the beginning probably has psychomotor delay, either from intrauterine or perinatal damage or from hereditary factors. On the other hand, a period of normal development, after which the child slows or regresses, suggests the onset of a recent or acquired problem such as seizures, meningitis, encephalitis or lead poisoning.

Many neurologic disorders are familial, including some types of epilepsy, migraine headaches and certain tumors. Therefore, specific questions about family history are essential. Often parents will omit information, thinking it unrelated or unimportant. The neurologist should inquire whether any family member (even distantly related) has had seizures,

The Neurologic Examination

headaches, weakness, gait problems, mental retardation, learning disorders or psychiatric problems. A history of other disorders that are not directly of a neurologic nature but which can affect the nervous system secondarily must also be sought; among these are thyroid disease, high blood pressure and diabetes.

Questions about the pregnancy and delivery may also add information about the child's problem. Did the mother take medication or did she have any infections during the pregnancy? Was she exposed to rubella (German measles)? Did the baby breathe immediately after delivery? The child's previous illnesses should be recorded in detail. Meningitis, encephalitis, severe head trauma, lead ingestion and many other disorders can cause long-lasting neurologic problems.

After a thorough history is completed, an equally extensive examination is begun. A general physical examination is carried out first with a check of the eyes, ears, nose, throat, heart, lungs, abdomen, genitalia and limbs. Often neurologic problems, especially those of a hereditary or developmental nature, are associated with abnormalities in other systems as well, such as heart murmurs, low-set or malformed ears. Any unusual pigmentation of the skin should also be noted.

The mental status of the patient then is evaluated. Is he alert and attentive? Does the child respond to verbal commands, follow directions appropriately for age? Does he have age-appropriate skills, e.g., does he recognize colors, stack blocks, copy figures, draw a person, name familiar objects? If the child is of school age, tests of spelling, math, reading and writing are given.

Functions of major areas of the brain then are tested in a systematic way (see Fig. 1–1).

Evaluation of cranial nerves is performed next (Table 2–1). Can the child see, hear, smell adequately? Do the eyes, facial muscles, mouth and tongue move properly? Is speech clear and articulation of sounds appropriate for age?

Deep tendon reflexes are tested by tapping the tendon (e.g., at the knee) and causing stretch of the appropriate muscle, resulting in a visible movement (leg, knee jerk). In children,

TABLE 2-1.—THE CRANIAL NERVES

NAME	FUNCTION
Olfactory	Smell
Optic	Vision
Oculomotor	Movement of eye muscles; pupil dilation
Trochlear	Movement of eye outward and downward
Trigeminal	Sensation to cornea and face; movement of muscles used in chewing
Abducens	Movement of eye laterally (outward)
Facial	Movement of facial muscles; taste in anterior two-thirds of tongue
Acoustic	Hearing and equilibrium
Glossopharyngeal	Taste in posterior one-third of tongue; movement of pharynx; sensation to pharynx and soft palate
Vagus	Movement of pharynx and larynx; sensation to pharynx and larynx
Spinal accessory	Movement of pharynx, uvula and palate; rotation of head (sternocleidomastoid muscle) and elevation of shoulders (trapezius muscle)
Hypoglossal	Movement of tongue

reflexes usually are brisk and should be symmetric. Asymmetric responses or a marked increase or decrease in reflex activity may be significant.

The Babinski sign is checked. This test is performed by stroking the bottom of the foot from the outside of the heel forward and curving over the ball of the foot with an object such as the examiner's fingernail or a key. The big toe flexes or moves downward in a normal (negative) response; the big toe extends or goes up and other toes fan out in a positive Babinski sign. The Babinski sign is normal in infants up to the age of 12–18 months. A positive Babinski after this age may indicate spasticity. However, one must be careful to distinguish a positive response from voluntary withdrawal by a sensitive child.

Muscle tone is evaluated by the examiner moving the arms and legs of the patient gently. Tone is the amount of contraction in a muscle at rest. Normally there is a small amount of resistance to passive movements, which is easily overcome. Too much resistance indicates hypertonia (increased muscle tone) and may be related to spasticity; too little resistance suggests hypotonia (decreased muscle tone) and may be associated with muscle disorders or cerebellar dysfunction.

Cerebral dominance may be of importance in evaluating possible neurologic dysfunction. Hand, eye and foot preference are noted by the examiner. Which hand does the child use to reach for objects or to draw or write? Which foot does the child use to kick a ball? When given a "telescope" of rolled-up paper to look through, which eye does the child choose? These maneuvers tell us not only if the child has right or left hemispheric dominance but, more important, if there is mixed dominance; that is, does the child prefer his left hand and right foot or vice versa? Mixed dominance may be an indication of cerebral dysfunction and appears to be more commonly associated with learning disabilities than is pure right or left dominance.

At the same time, coordination is tested. This part of the examination may be performed in a variety of ways, depending on the patient's age and ability to cooperate. For example, a small child may be asked to reach for or stack blocks. This maneuver demonstrates not only an age-appropriate skill but can also elicit abnormalities, e.g., poor grasp, tremor of the hand or arm or dysmetria. Dysmetria, or pastpointing, is present if, when reaching for an object, the patient misses the target and reaches past it. Coordination can also be tested by having the patient pat his hand on his knee, tap his toe on the floor repeatedly or touch his index finger to the finger of the examiner and then back to his nose. The ability to coordinate such movements depends on an intact cerebellum.

Sensation probably is the most difficult modality to examine in a child. However, this is quite important and should not be omitted because of the child's age or poor cooperation. Sensation can be tested in a variety of ways. The least complicated is to tickle the arm or leg and to watch for withdrawal. Intact sensation may also be evaluated by using a sharp object such as a pin and again noting withdrawal of the appropriate extremity. In the more cooperative child, however, more specific testing can be performed. For instance, a vibrating tuning fork can be placed on the child's wrist or knee and the patient asked to tell the examiner when the vibration or "buzzing sound" stops. Surprisingly, even small children can respond to this examination properly if they are relaxed and not fearful.

Sensation of light touch can be examined by asking the child to close his eyes and then point to the place where the examiner has just touched him. If the examination has been performed in such a way that the child feels comfortable with the examiner and believes, in fact, that he is playing a game, it is not difficult to perform an adequate sensory examination.

Motor skills are evaluated extensively as part of the neurologic examination. Muscle bulk is checked for atrophy (decrease in size) or hypertrophy (increase in size). The child is asked to walk, run, hop on one foot, skip and walk heel to toe "as though he is walking a tightrope." To check a Romberg sign, he then is asked to stand with his feet together and to close his eyes. A normal person can stand in this position without difficulty; a patient with cerebellar dysfunction or with absence of position sense will fall to one side when the eyes are closed. This is considered a positive Romberg. In testing gait, one looks for a limp or other asymmetry between the two legs, lack of arm swing and poor balance. These are all indications of possible central nervous system dysfunction.

Any involuntary movements should be carefully characterized. These include the following:

Myoclonic jerks—brief, irregular contractions of muscles.
Tremors—rapid, irregular, "shaky" movements of body segments (e.g., hands, head).
Athetosis—irregular, wandering or writhing movements, usually of fingers or toes.
Chorea—coarse, jerky movements involving larger segments of the body (e.g., arms, legs).
Dystonia—slow, twisting or writhing movements of limbs or trunk.

The autonomic nervous system is evaluated by checking for bladder distention, tone of rectal sphincter muscles, color and temperature of skin and ability to perspire.

In examining an infant, the developmental reflexes described in Chapter 1 (tonic neck reflex, Moro reflex, etc.) should be tested. Head control, that is, the ability of the infant to hold his head erect, should be evaluated carefully by several methods. The examiner first holds the infant's hands and pulls him from a lying to a sitting position, noting whether the head lags behind the trunk (Fig. 2–1). This maneuver is called

The Neurologic Examination

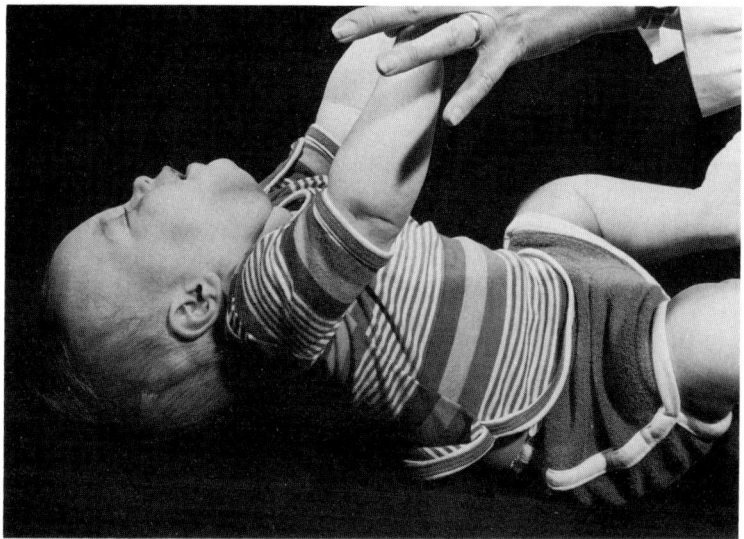

Fig. 2–1.—A 10-month-old infant with cerebral palsy demonstrating poor head control while being lifted from supine position.

the *traction* response. Normal infants after about 4 months of age should have no head lag. The examiner then places the infant in a prone position (face down) and observes his ability to lift his head off the table. At 1 month, an infant should be able to lift his head off the table and at 3 months his head and chest.

An infant should be observed for stability of the body while sitting (supported if necessary). The examiner should also hold the baby by the trunk and stand him up to see if he can support weight on his legs.

In infants under 1 year of age, transillumination of the head is a useful test that is performed by holding the lighted end of a flashlight against the child's head in a darkened room. The infant's skull is thin, and any abnormal accumulation of fluid around the brain may result in an increased spread of light in that region.

With a stethoscope, the physician listens to the child's head for abnormal noises, called *bruits*, which may be present in normal infants but may also indicate that blood vessels are enlarged or malformed. If an infant has an unusually large head, the examiner should tap the head lightly with the fingers and listen for a "cracked-pot" sound (Macewen's sign), which suggests the presence of increased pressure inside the head.

If the clinical history suggests the possibility of a seizure disorder, the child then is asked to hyperventilate. That is, he is asked to take several deep breaths over a 2–3-minute period while being observed closely by the examiner. Hyperventilation frequently brings out petit mal seizures in children who have this type of seizure disorder. Petit mal or absence seizures are characterized by brief periods during which activity stops, the child stares into space and, at times, his eyelids flutter. These last no longer than about 15–30 seconds and can easily be missed unless the examiner is aware of the manifestations of this type of seizure disorder.

What conclusions can be reached from the neurologic examination described? By having evaluated age-appropriate skills in the child, a developmental quotient (DQ), which is the per cent of assessed developmental age (DA) measured against the chronologic age (CA), can be derived. Thus, $DQ = DA/CA \times 100$. For example, if an 8-year-old child performs at only a 4-year level, his developmental quotient is 50. The average developmental quotient for a normal child is 100. Therefore, the child with a developmental quotient of 50 might be functioning in the retarded range. On the other hand, a child may function appropriately for age in most areas but may have a specific learning disability. For instance, the child may not be able to read (dyslexia) or may have difficulty with math (dyscalculia) while performing all other skills properly. This child should not be classified as retarded or mentally delayed, but as having a specific learning disability. Spasticity, weakness and difficulty with coordination or balance can all be diagnosed from the neurologic examination. Hyperactive behavior can also be recognized. Certain hereditary diseases that have characteristic findings, for instance, Down's syndrome (mongolism), can be readily recognized in the process of the examination.

After conclusions are reached, the neurologist may make certain recommendations. Further testing may be necessary. X-rays of the head, an electroencephalogram (EEG or brain wave test) or computerized x-ray of the brain (CT scan) are all useful diagnostic aids. An EEG is helpful in detecting possible seizure disorders. A CT scan (Fig. 2–2) might be indicated if structural abnormalities are suspected; that is, a brain tumor, vascular malformation or cyst in the brain.

Special classes may be recommended; for example, learning disabilities groups for children with a specific learning disorder or classes for the educable mentally handicapped for a child who is functioning in the retarded range. Medication may be recommended. Children with seizure disorders may need long-term anticonvulsant therapy; those with pathologically hyperactive behavior may benefit from medication to reduce the hyperactivity. Rehabilitative therapy may be indicated; a speech, occupational or physical therapist may be

Fig. 2–2.—Normal computerized tomographic scan. *1*, bones of skull; *2*, brain substance; *3*, ventricles; *4*, orbits of eyes.

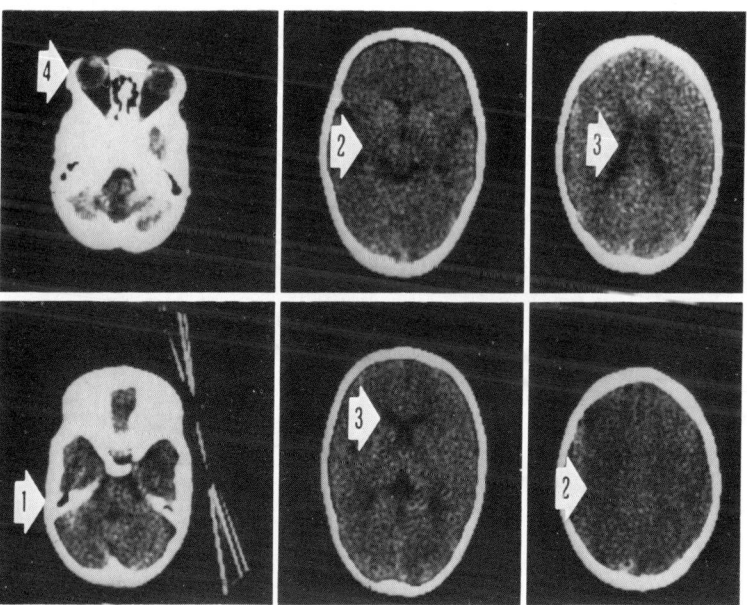

helpful in implementing therapy designed to improve the child's performance. Orthopedic aids such as braces, special lifts in the shoes or similar devices may be necessary. In rare cases, surgery may be necessary to correct the problem. For example, children with brain tumors or some structural malformations in the brain or spinal cord may benefit from surgical correction of the abnormality. Similarly, children with spasticity may have marked contractures ("freezing") of the joints, which can be surgically corrected for better range of motion of the involved joint.

In summary, the comprehensive neurologic examination evaluates all aspects of central and peripheral nervous system function and is potentially of significant benefit to the child who suffers from a previously unrecognized neurologic disorder.

3

SEIZURE DISORDERS

THE WORD *epilepsy* is derived from the Greek *epilēpsia*, meaning seizure. In neurologic practice, the word is used to specify *recurrent* seizures or convulsions. A seizure may be defined as a transient disturbance in brain function caused by an interruption in normal electrical activity in the brain that manifests itself as some alteration of consciousness or of sensory or motor activity. Seizures may be generalized, that is, causing loss of consciousness, or focal, causing alteration of sensation or muscle function in parts of the body, with preservation of awareness.

Seizures are not uncommon occurrences in childhood. An estimated 3–5% of all children will have at least one seizure by the age of 5 years. Most of these occur in the presence of high fever and do not constitute epilepsy. Epilepsy is not a disease but a symptom of underlying neurologic dysfunction. In some patients, the underlying cause can be identified (Table 3–1). In the majority, however, no identifiable cause can be determined, and the patient is said to have "idiopathic" epilepsy. *In general,* children with symptomatic epilepsy in whom the underlying disease is not correctable tend

TABLE 3–1.—CAUSES OF SYMPTOMATIC EPILEPSY

Hereditary (e.g., familial myoclonus, petit mal epilepsy)
Malformations of brain development
Birth injury
Head trauma
Infectious diseases (encephalitis, meningitis)
Mass lesions (tumor, brain abscess, blood vessel malformation)
Degenerative diseases of the nervous system (e.g., Tay-Sachs)
Metabolic abnormalities (e.g., vitamin B_6 deficiency or dependency)
Toxins (lead poisoning)

TABLE 3-2.—TYPES OF SEIZURES

I. Generalized
  A. Grand mal
  B. Petit mal
  C. Psychomotor
  D. Akinetic
  E. Infantile spasms
II. Focal
  A. Motor
  B. Sensory
  C. Adversive
  D. Segmental myoclonus
III. Febrile

to have more severe seizure disorders than those with correctable causes or with the idiopathic form.

Seizures are characterized clinically by the type of activity that they produce. Manifestations of seizures are extremely varied, and for purposes of clarity only representative descriptions of common seizure types will be presented here (Table 3-2).

GENERALIZED SEIZURES

GRAND MAL.—This type of seizure usually occurs without warning, although the child may show some indication, such as irritability, personality change or clumsiness, for minutes or hours prior to the seizure. At the onset of the episode, eyes may roll up or deviate to one side, loss of consciousness occurs and tonic (stiffening) or clonic (jerking) movements of the arms and legs begin. Muscle contractions may be so severe as to interfere with breathing, and the child may turn blue or stop breathing entirely. Muscles of the jaw also tighten and if the tongue is caught between clenched jaws, lacerations can occur. As the attack subsides, movements become less violent and finally stop. Loss of bladder and/or bowel control can occur during the attack. Sometimes vomiting is seen as well. Following the cessation of seizure activity, the child may go to sleep or remain confused or stuporous for several hours.

In epileptic children, several factors have been identified

GENERALIZED SEIZURES

that may precipitate seizures. These include fatigue, stress, fever, hyperventilation or prolonged deep breathing and some medications. These things should be judiciously avoided in children with seizure disorders.

PETIT MAL. — This type of seizure has its usual onset in children between the ages of 5 and 10. Such spells are extremely subtle and can easily be missed, with the child appearing to be merely inattentive or "daydreaming." Onset is abrupt, with a brief lapse of consciousness (5–10 seconds) and little or no loss of body tone, so that the child does not fall down. Eyelid twitching and lip-smacking movements may be observed as the only motor manifestation of the seizure. After the attack, the child resumes normal activities immediately and is unaware of this brief lapse of consciousness. Petit mal seizures are quite frequent and may occur numerous times a day.

PSYCHOMOTOR SEIZURES. — This type of seizure results from irritation of a specific area of the brain — the temporal lobe — and may assume a wide variety of clinical features. In general, the spell may be heralded by an aura consisting of a strange sensation; for example, an odd odor or a visual or auditory hallucination. There is then a sudden alteration of awareness accompanied by stereotyped and sometimes complex activity; for example, repetitive verbal responses, singing or movements such as picking at clothes. At times, these symptoms are followed by grand mal seizures as well. After the spell there typically is some residual confusion for several minutes to hours and amnesia for the seizure itself.

AKINETIC SEIZURES ("drop attacks"). — This type of spell consists of a very brief loss of muscle tone, resulting in a sometimes violent fall to the ground, accompanied by momentary loss of consciousness. Afterward, the child immediately resumes normal activity. However, injuries are common with this type of seizure because of the force with which the child may fall down and the lack of warning.

INFANTILE SPASMS (massive myoclonic seizures of infancy). — This type of seizure usually occurs in infants between 5 and 10 months of age; it rarely is seen in older children. Each episode is brief and consists of a sudden jerk or twitch involving the whole body. At times, the infant appears to flex arms, legs and head briefly and simultaneously. An irritable cry may accompany the movement. These spells recur in clusters many times a day.

FOCAL SEIZURES

MOTOR.—These spells are localized, usually jerking or stiffening movements of one part of the body; for example, an arm or a leg. The child maintains awareness of his surroundings but cannot voluntarily stop the seizure activity. The movements may remain localized or spread to involve other parts of the body. In some instances, the seizure eventually becomes generalized and the child loses consciousness.

SENSORY.—This attack also is localized but it is characterized by onset of some sensory symptom; for example, a feeling of tingling or numbness in one part of the body. This type of seizure also may spread to other parts of the body and become generalized.

ADVERSIVE.—In this type of seizure, the head and eyes suddenly deviate to one side. Although the child may remain awake, he cannot control head and eye movements during the attack.

SEGMENTAL MYOCLONUS.—This is a sudden, single, brief jerk or twitch of a body part, for example, arm or leg, without loss of consciousness or other manifestations of seizure activity. These may recur many times a day and may be the result of spinal cord or localized central nervous system abnormalities.

FEBRILE SEIZURES

A subclassification of seizure types is that of "benign febrile convulsions" (Table 3-3). This entity is responsible for the majority of single seizures in children under 4 years of age. The cause is not known, although such seizures are known to

TABLE 3-3.—CHARACTERISTICS OF
"BENIGN FEBRILE CONVULSIONS"

Age occurrence 6 months to 4 years
Temperature greater than 102°
Brief duration—less than 15 minutes
Generalized without focal features
EEG normal 2 weeks later
Family history of similar episodes positive in 50% of patients

have a familial incidence. Onset usually is between the ages of 6 months and 4 years, and seizures typically occur as the fever suddenly rises in a child with a viral infection (for example, roseola or an upper respiratory infection). These seizures are brief in duration and generalized without focal features. The electroencephalogram in such children is normal within 1 month after the episode. The primary concern about recurrent febrile seizures is that they may produce an irritative focus in the brain that will lead to future afebrile seizures.

ELECTROENCEPHALOGRAPHY

The EEG is a useful diagnostic test for many types of neurologic problems and may be particularly helpful in patients with seizure disorders. This test is performed by placing a series of small metal electrodes on the scalp at specified positions over the head (Fig. 3-1). The electrodes are connected by wires to a series of amplifiers, which, in turn, are connected to a polygraph that records the brain's electrical activity detected by these electrodes onto a sheet of paper. In this way, the patterns of electrical activity over the brain's surface can be examined (Fig. 3-2). Normal activity during waking and at different stages of sleep is known, and, therefore, abnormalities in these patterns can be detected. Several types of abnormal electrical activity can occur. These include abnormal and excessive slowing of activity and unusually fast and sharp activity. Many people with seizure disorders will have spike discharges on the EEG (Fig. 3-3). These suggest that there is an "irritation" (such as a scar) in the brain. Such information may be helpful in determining the type of seizure that the pa-

26 Seizure Disorders

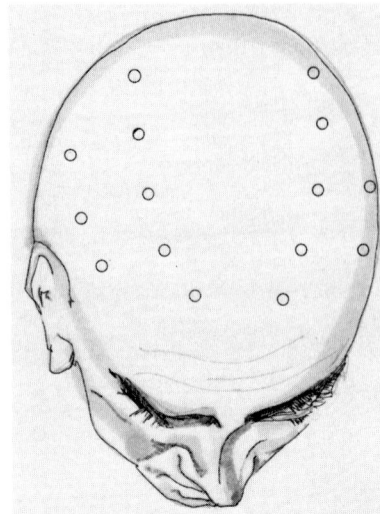

Fig. 3–1.—Placement of electrodes for recording electroencephalogram.

Fig. 3–2.—Segment of electroencephalogram during sleep in a 3-year-old; normal tracing.

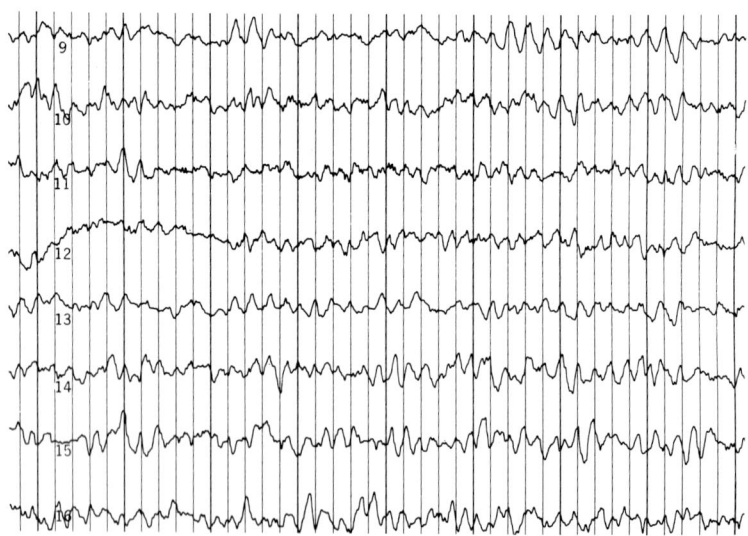

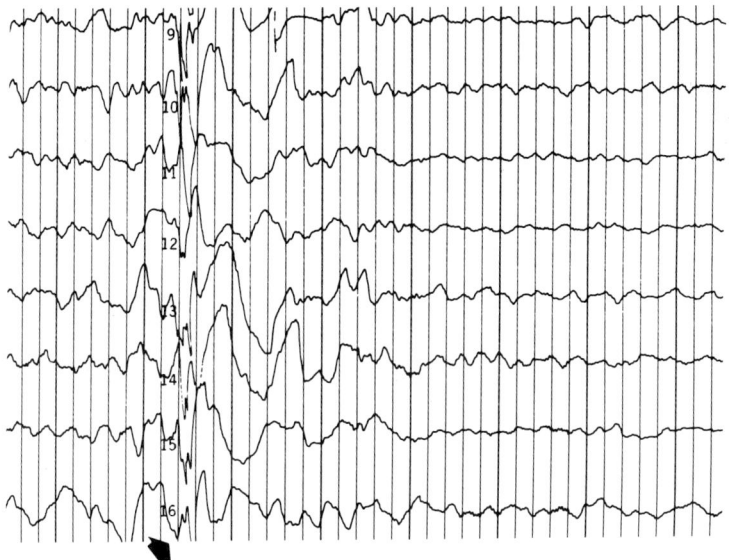

Fig. 3-3.—Abnormal EEG during sleep in a 3-year-old; generalized spike and wave discharge recorded *(arrow)*.

tient is experiencing and the area of brain involved in the case of focal seizures.

However, the EEG is merely an adjunct to diagnosis and is not to be used as the sole criterion for treatment of a patient. For example, a small percentage of the "normal" population, that is, those in whom no seizure activity has ever occurred, will have abnormal EEGs. On the other hand, approximately 40% of children who have documented seizure disorders will have a normal EEG. Thus, the EEG can be used only in conjunction with the clinical history and response of the patient to medication.

TREATMENT OF SEIZURE DISORDERS

Treatment is based on an attempt to minimize the irritable focus in the brain and prevent the spread of abnormal electrical discharges. This is accomplished through various anticonvulsant medications. The aim of therapy is to prevent further seizures entirely whenever possible. Therefore, anticonvulsant medications must be taken daily, sometimes over the course of several years. Once a child has been seizure-free for a minimum of 2 years, the medication can be gradually discontinued and in many cases seizures will not recur. Most children do not require lifelong medication.

Probably the most frequently prescribed anticonvulsant is phenobarbital, which is effective for many types of seizure disorders. It is most effective for grand mal convulsions. Phenobarbital is a long-acting barbiturate and because of its length of action does not cause psychologic dependence, as may some of the shorter-acting barbiturates. Occasional allergic reactions occur with phenobarbital in the form of a rash or lymph node enlargement. In these cases, the medication should be discontinued promptly. Drowsiness is reported infrequently and may disappear after the child has become accustomed to the medication. The most common side effect is hyperactive behavior and short attention span, at times so prominent as to warrant discontinuing the drug. This type of behavior often interferes with schoolwork and interpersonal relations. In these patients, another medication should be substituted. Phenobarbital never should be stopped abruptly, because doing so may precipitate a seizure. Rather, it should be tapered slowly according to a program set up by the physician.

Mephobarbital (Mebaral) is similar to phenobarbital but does not as commonly produce the side effect of hyperactivity. Therefore, it is used in children who have had adverse behavioral problems secondary to phenobarbital. The primary side effect of mephobarbital is drowsiness, which may subside after the child becomes accustomed to the medication.

Diphenylhydantoin (Dilantin, DPH) is also a commonly prescribed anticonvulsant and is most effective in grand mal seizure control. Allergic reactions may also occur with DPH and include rash, fever, lymph node enlargement and a hepatitis-like illness. In these instances, the drug should be stopped immediately and the physician notified. Possible side effects of DPH are numerous. Increased growth of hair on the body and increase in gum size may occur after long-term treatment and do not necessitate removal of the medication, although these cause cosmetic problems that may be distressing, especially in a young girl. Potentially more serious side effects are rare, but may include liver damage, bone marrow depression and elevations of blood sugar. It is imperative that a child on any medication be under close medical supervision and that such side effects be treated accordingly.

DPH may also inhibit vitamin D absorption into the body. Therefore, some patients may require additional vitamin supplements while taking this medication. In high doses, DPH may cause lethargy, unsteady gait and inability to concentrate. All of these symptoms might interfere with normal school performance and suggest that the dosage may need to be decreased.

Ethosuximide (Zarontin) is the usual treatment of choice for petit mal seizures and has some effectiveness in combination with other anticonvulsants in patients with mixed seizure disorders. Side effects of this drug include headaches and dizziness, which are rare. The primary complication of this medication is bone marrow depression, which may result in abnormally low levels of white and red blood cells. Although rare, this complication, when it occurs, can be serious. Therefore, children on chronic ethosuximide therapy should be followed carefully and blood counts checked periodically. If there is an indication that bone marrow depression has occurred, medication should be stopped promptly by the physician. With early detection, the problem usually is reversible.

Primidone (Mysoline) is used in the treatment of psychomotor seizures. This drug has an anticonvulsant action of its own but is also partially metabolized to phenobarbital. Because of this, there may be an additive effect in patients receiving both phenobarbital and primidone, and excessive drowsiness may occur. Side effects of primidone include drowsiness, irritability, slurring of speech and unsteady gait. The dose must be carefully adjusted by the physician to give maximal benefit and minimal side effects.

Three relatively new anticonvulsants now are in use in the United States and have been quite beneficial in treating complicated seizure disorders. Carbamazepine (Tegretol) is quite effective in psychomotor seizures particularly, although it is also beneficial in a variety of other types of convulsive disorders. This medication has little effect on the child's ability to function well in daily life. Side effects are rare and include nausea, vomiting, dizziness and double vision. Possible complications include bone marrow depression and liver damage. These problems, although rare with carbamazepine, are sufficiently serious that close medical supervision and frequent blood tests are necessary while the child is taking this drug.

Clonazepam (Clonopin) is effective in many types of convulsive disorders, particularly focal motor, akinetic and myoclonic seizures. It has also been used for petit mal epilepsy with some success. Unfortunately, clonazepam frequently causes drowsiness that may be sufficiently prominent to interfere with the child's school performance and cause a decrease in appetite. At times, this can be averted by beginning with extremely low doses. Other complications are minimal.

Sodium valproate has only quite recently been released for use in the United States. Side effects appear to be minimal except for the possibility of liver damage, and this medication apparently is quite effective in controlling many types of seizures.

ACTH is a corticosteroid hormone that has been useful in treating a specific type of seizure, that of massive myoclonic seizures of infancy, or infantile spasms. It is given by intramuscular injection daily for 6 weeks. Side effects include irritability, elevations of blood pressure, changes in appetite and excessive hair and fat distribution in the body. These effects usually reverse when ACTH is discontinued, and in selected patients this medication is extremely effective in seizure control.

Acetazolamide (Diamox) is not an anticonvulsant but sometimes is useful as an adjunct to therapy in combination with anticonvulsant medications. It is particularly helpful in mixed seizure disorders, which are difficult to control with one drug alone.

Some epileptic patients require combinations of several anticonvulsants simultaneously in order to completely control seizure activity. This is most properly carried out under close supervision of a pediatric neurologist who is familiar with anticonvulsant drug side effects and multiple drug interactions.

PROGNOSIS

The long-term outlook for patients with recurrent seizures is in part dependent on the underlying cause and in part on early detection and treatment. Thus, children in whom seizures are the result of severe brain injuries (e.g., anoxic damage) or developmental malformations of the brain will, in general, be more difficult to control adequately and may have lifelong seizure problems. On the other hand, the majority of seizure disorders are idiopathic, as mentioned earlier, and respond well to anticonvulsant therapy. These children may have complete seizure control and lead normal lives. This is the primary aim of anticonvulsant therapy. The usual length of treatment for seizure disorders is 2-4 years. If no seizures have occurred in that time, medication can usually be discontinued safely.

PRECAUTIONS FOR CHILDREN WITH RECURRENT SEIZURES

Epileptic children suffer at least as much from the social stigma of epilepsy as from the seizure disorder itself. Such children usually are normal in every way except for having seizures and should be treated as normal healthy children. A few precautions obviously must be taken to prevent serious injury if the child has a seizure. Aside from these, however, the child should be encouraged to engage in age-appropriate activities of interest to him and not be overly protected to the point of social isolation.

Appropriate precautions include the following:

1. Do not swim without a competent person, knowledgeable in lifesaving techniques, in constant attendance; do not bathe in a bathtub without supervision.
2. Do not climb in high, unprotected places (e.g., "jungle gyms").
3. Do not work with heavy machinery or hot electrical appliances.
4. Do not drive a vehicle.

Aside from these limitations, the child should be encouraged to work and play normally and should be expected to assume the normal age-appropriate responsibilities that are required of all children. Also, the presence of a seizure disorder should not be cause for lack of appropriate discipline for the child, since this will encourage the idea that the child is "different" and immune to normal social restraints.

MANAGEMENT OF A SEIZURE

A seizure can be very frightening to watch, especially for the first time, but it is essential to remain calm in order to help the child who is having a seizure. Procedures to follow if a child has a seizure include the following:

1. Remain calm!
2. Lay the child down, preferably on the floor, so that he cannot fall or bump into any object; move all sharp objects out of the way.
3. Turn head and body to one side.
4. Do not place fingers or any other object in the child's mouth.
5. Do not restrain the child (tight restraints during a seizure can result in fractured bones).
6. Remove any tight clothing (necktie, scarf).
7. Do not give the child anything to drink during the seizure and do not throw water on him.
8. Observe details of the motor components of the seizure in order to later report these to appropriate medical personnel or parents.
9. When the seizure is over, allow the child to rest and call the physician for further instruction, if indicated.

4

HEADACHES IN CHILDREN

THE PROBLEM OF HEADACHES in childhood has received little attention in the medical literature. However, it has been estimated that as many as 60-75% of children have complained of significant headaches by the age of 15 years. Children, especially under the age of 8, do not commonly develop headaches that are primarily psychosomatic or hysterical. Therefore, if a child complains of such symptoms, a thorough neurologic evaluation is indicated. Classification of headaches in children is given in Table 4-1.

MIGRAINE HEADACHES

This type of vascular headache is not uncommon in children, occurring with an incidence of 2-5% in childhood. There is a strong familial incidence of migraine; that is, a child with this complaint often will have siblings, parents or other relatives with similar problems. There is also an increased incidence of migraine headaches occurring in families in which seizure disorders are present.

Vascular headaches, including migraine, occur because of sudden and excessive widening or dilation of blood vessels inside the head. This accounts for most of the symptoms that patients with migraine headaches describe. Migraine headaches are intermittent and occur suddenly and unpredictably. Frequently they occur on only one side of the head, although, in children, the localization may be indistinct. They are associated most often with nausea and vomiting and sometimes with transient visual or other localized neurologic deficits. The migraine attack can be divided into three phases:

TABLE 4-1.—CLASSIFICATION OF
HEADACHES IN CHILDREN

I. Vascular headaches
   A. Simple migraine
   B. Complicated migraine
   C. Cluster headaches
II. Nonvascular headaches
   A. Tension-muscular
   B. Depression
   C. Sinus
   D. Secondary to eye and dental problems
III. Post-traumatic headaches
IV. Headaches as a result of underlying neurologic disease
   A. Tumor
   B. Pseudotumor cerebri
   C. Meningitis and encephalitis
   D. Psychomotor seizures
   E. Encephalopathies with increased intracranial pressure

---

1. Preheadache phase (prodrome). During this phase, sudden constriction of blood vessels in the head takes place. When this occurs, preheadache symptoms (auras) appear and may include such problems as visual disturbances—for example, flashing lights or zigzag lines may appear in the patient's field of vision—speech difficulties, dizziness, weakness, and mood changes.

2. Headache phase. During this phase, excessive widening or dilation of the blood vessels inside the head occurs. This causes a throbbing or pounding headache that may be associated with nausea and vomiting.

3. Late headache phase. During this time, the walls of the dilated blood vessels become swollen and rigid. The headache then changes from pounding to dull and the scalp overlying the headache area may feel tender to the touch.

Postmigraine head or neck pain may result from tension placed on muscles during the initial headache phase.

The cause of migraine still is obscure. Hereditary and familial factors appear to play a role. The syndrome has also been linked with allergies—for example, to a substance in cheese called tyramine—and to epilepsy. However, the relationship of migraine to epilepsy is poorly understood.

The symptoms of migraine in childhood are not as typical as

Migraine Headaches

those in adults. The headache often is poorly localized and may even occur all over the head. In young children, the only evidence of headache may be that the child lets out a cry and grabs his head until the headache is over. Vomiting is common, as is sensitivity to light (photophobia) and to sound (phonophobia). Headaches can be induced by stress, flickering lights, lack of sleep and irregular eating habits. Migraine headaches usually last from a few minutes to a few hours, but rarely longer than 2-3 hours for each individual headache. The frequency varies and they may occur as often as once a day or as seldom as once a year. The child usually wants to lie down until the headache is over. Migraine headaches can occur at any age and are seen even in very young children.

With complicated migraine, other symptoms are associated with the headache. They may include weakness of one side of the body (hemiplegic migraine), and difficulty with eye movements and widening of the pupils (ophthalmoplegic migraine). These symptoms usually disappear when the headache subsides.

One treatment of migraine in childhood, based on the suspected relationship of migraine to epilepsy, is anticonvulsant medication similar to that used to treat seizure disorders. The most commonly used medications in this class include phenobarbital, methobarbital, diphenylhydantoin and carbamazepine. Side effects of these medications are discussed in Chapter 3. The doses used for treatment of migraine usually are lower than those for treatment of epilepsy. Medication is given daily for 3-6 months to prevent further headaches.

Other medications used in childhood migraine include ergotamines, which act by narrowing the blood vessels. However, there are three problems encountered with this type of medication. The most significant drawback is that, to work effectively, ergotamines should be taken as soon as the prodromal symptoms appear. Many children do not have a prodrome before the headache begins, while others are unable to tell their parents soon enough to make the medication effective. The second problem is that some children have a very prominent preheadache phase to the migraine, during which the blood vessels narrow abruptly. In these cases one would not want to use a medication that would further narrow the blood vessels and produce more severe symptoms. The third problem is that ergots have many potentially harmful side effects because of their action on narrowing the blood vessels. These include nausea and vomiting, sweating, weakness, muscle pain, numbness and tingling in the hands and feet, chest pain and changes in heart rate. Excessive use can cause more serious side effects, e.g., from blockage of blood supply to the hands and feet. These side effects are not frequent but are serious enough to warrant close supervision of a patient who is being treated with this medication.

A third medication that is used in treatment of migraine, very infrequently in children, is methysergide. This drug modifies the blood vessels so that they do not open and close to the degree that typically occurs with migraine. This medication is useful when the more common drugs are ineffective and when the headaches are extremely frequent, because it prevents further headaches from occurring. It must be taken daily for 6 weeks. Prolonged use of methysergide has been linked with a very rare but potentially severe side effect called retroperitoneal fibrosis. In this condition, fibrous bands form around organs such as the kidneys and can cause disturbance of function in these organs. For this reason, methysergide should not be used over long periods. Again, treatment should be carefully monitored by the physician.

For mild migraine symptoms, aspirin, acetaminophen and combinations of mild pain relievers can be used for symptomatic relief.

The outlook for childhood migraine is good. Many children with such headaches will have disappearance of symptoms during or after puberty and may be headache-free for many years. Migraine may or may not recur in adult life.

CLUSTER HEADACHES

This type of headache is extremely rare in childhood. The youngest child reported in the medical literature had cluster headaches at 11 years of age. This form usually occurs in middle age and in men more often than in women. The cause is not known, but evidence points to a sudden discharge into the blood stream of a chemical called histamine, which causes widening of the blood vessels in the head.

The characteristic symptoms associated with this type of headache include sudden onset, with occurrence in clusters; that is, each headache may last for only a few hours but the headaches recur frequently for several weeks to months, after which they may disappear for some length of time and then recur periodically. The headache itself is characterized by severe, sharp, pounding pain over one side of the head. This is accompanied by flushing of the face, tearing of the eye and congestion of the nostril on the same side of the face as the pain. Unlike migraine, there is no prodromal or preheadache warning phase. The headaches often occur more frequently at night and may awaken the patient from sleep. Symptoms begin abruptly and cease just as abruptly. Vomiting accompanying the head pain rarely is a feature of this condition. Attacks can be precipitated by drinking alcoholic beverages.

Treatment consists of a trial of one of the ergot preparations. If this fails, a course of methysergide may be given for a period of 4-6 weeks. Patients should be warned to avoid anything known to precipitate these headaches, such as alcohol.

TENSION HEADACHES

As the name implies, tension headaches occur after prolonged tension or sustained contraction of neck and scalp muscles; for example, during anxiety or fear. The headache typically begins after the tension is eased and the patient begins to relax.

The typical features of tension headaches include slow onset of discomfort with no prodromal or preheadache phase. The pain may last for several hours to several days; it usually is felt all over the head, is nonpulsating and rarely is accompanied by nausea or vomiting. This type of pain may be a secondary accompaniment to other headaches, such as migraine. Often these headaches do not interfere with the patient's daily activities. Treatment consists of mild analgesics such as aspirin or acetaminophen. If muscle tension is excessive, diazepam or caffeine may be useful.

DEPRESSION HEADACHES

These are closely related to the pain secondary to tension and are associated with chronic anxiety and depression. This type of pain has a slow onset and no preheadache phase. It is described characteristically as a band-like pressure around the head. Treatment for this type of problem includes mild analgesics symptomatically, but the real treatment is to determine the cause of underlying depression and to try to remove that. Children are not immune to periods of depression any more than are adults, and depression should not be overlooked as a possible cause of childhood headaches.

SINUS HEADACHES

This type of problem is common with acute sinus infections but can also be associated with long-term inflammation of the sinuses. Headache may be the most prominent symptom of a recent sinus infection. At times, the pain may be referred elsewhere in the head, but usually it is present in areas adjacent to the inflamed sinus and is associated with tenderness over that area. The characteristics of sinus headaches include gradual onset with variable duration, at times as long as the inflammation persists. The pain is described as deep, dull and aching and is associated with tenderness to touch over the sinus area. The pain is intensified by stooping, coughing, head-down position or any jarring of the person. Treatment for this type of problem includes decongestants, mild analgesics, if necessary, and antibiotics if an active infection is present.

Head pain can occur as a result of dental problems such as gum infections and tooth abscesses. This type of pain usually is dull and aching and sometimes is localized over the jaw but at times radiates to other parts of the head. "Eye strain" can also cause headaches that are primarily due to muscle tension. Both of these problems are treated by appropriate dental and ophthalmologic consultations.

POST-TRAUMATIC HEADACHES

Generalized or localized headaches frequently follow head injury. Such an injury may be mild, causing no immediate problem, or severe, such as concussion, producing a brief loss of consciousness. In many cases, no detectable brain damage has occurred, and the cause of such headaches is obscure. However, they may last from days to months after the original trauma. These headaches usually are constant, may be sharp or dull and are self-limited; that is, they gradually disappear with or without treatment. Children with previous emotional disturbances are particularly susceptible to prolonged post-traumatic headaches. The treatment for such problems is mild analgesics as indicated by the severity of the pain.

There is no reason for undue concern at the development of headaches after mild head injury, so long as the headache is the only symptom that the child exhibits. Other accompanying complaints would be of more concern; for example, arm or leg weakness, double vision or blurred vision. In children with significant head trauma such as a concussion, special x-ray studies (e.g., computerized tomography) may be performed to eliminate the possibility of a blood clot inside the head.

HEADACHES AS A RESULT OF UNDERLYING NEUROLOGIC DISEASE

A very small percentage of children with complaints of headaches have an underlying neurologic problem as the cause. However, since headaches can occur in the presence of structural and infectious brain disorders, they should be considered in the child with such complaints.

Headaches are common at some stage in the development of brain tumor growth. Such pain usually is intermittent, at least in the early stages, and is typically diffuse, occurring all over the head, although rarely the pain is localized over the tumor. The typical time of occurrence is in the morning, when the child first awakes, and at times is associated with forceful vomiting unpreceded by nausea. The headaches tend to get better as the morning goes on. This type of headache is a result of increased pressure inside the brain from the mass effect of the tumor.

Underlying brain tumor should be considered in the differential diagnosis of a patient with recurrent morning headaches, especially with associated vomiting. A thorough neurologic examination should be performed on such children to determine if further special x-ray studies should be obtained to look for the presence of a tumor.

One poorly understood and fortunately rare cause of headaches in children is a syndrome called *pseudotumor cerebri*. This is a condition in which brain swelling occurs, usually for no known reason. It has been associated with excessive intake of vitamins, with tetracycline and rarely with other medications. However, for most cases, no cause is found.

Symptoms include headache, which usually is generalized, vomiting and swelling of the optic nerve in the back of the eye. Diagnosis is made by eliminating other causes of brain swelling, such as infection and real tumor. Treatment consists of repeated spinal taps, which remove some of the spinal fluid and relieve pressure on the brain. At times, steroid hormone treatment is helpful in reducing pressure. This condition usually resolves in a period of weeks to months, after which the patient is free from symptoms. Occasionally, pseudotumor may be recurrent.

The primary complication of this condition is blindness from prolonged pressure on the optic nerve. Therefore, the child should be followed closely by a neurologist as well as by an ophthalmologist to determine if there is any compromise to visual acuity.

Infections of the brain (encephalitis) and surrounding coverings (meningitis) may produce headache as a result of increased pressure on the brain or from localized irritation. These headaches usually are severe, constant and generalized. A stiff neck, fever, nausea, vomiting, irritability and drowsiness may accompany the other symptoms. When these symptoms are present along with a headache, meningitis and encephalitis must be considered as possible diagnoses.

Occasionally, certain types of seizure disorders (notably psychomotor seizures) may be accompanied by headache

Headaches & Underlying Neurologic Disease

symptoms. This can be determined from the pattern of headaches and the presence of seizures in the patient; at times, an electroencephalogram is helpful in the diagnosis of this problem.

Metabolic and toxic derangements such as lead poisoning, hepatitis and Reye's syndrome can cause brain swelling, and headache may be an early symptom of encephalopathy.

The evaluation of headaches in children consists, first of all, of a complete history and thorough neurologic examination, including careful examination of the eyes. In general, an evaluation of headaches might include x-rays of the head and sinuses, an electroencephalogram and routine blood studies. Specific findings, such as tenderness over the sinuses, suggest that sinus x-rays should be obtained. A spinal tap would be indicated if the headaches had a sudden onset and were associated with fever and stiff neck. If a mass lesion such as a tumor or bleeding into the head is suspected, a special x-ray study called a computerized tomogram of the head should be obtained. These studies are not indicated in all children with headaches. The history and physical examination are the two most important components of the evaluation in a child who presents with headache symptoms.

5

STRUCTURAL DISEASES OF THE NERVOUS SYSTEM

DURING THE COURSE OF embryonic development, many intricate steps in cell migration, aggregation and specialization take place to form a complete human fetus. Because these steps are so complex there exists the possibility of mistakes occurring during every stage of development. These errors may result in abnormalities in the structure of the nervous system. Developmental and structural defects of the nervous system will be the subject of this chapter.

CEREBRAL MALFORMATIONS

ANENCEPHALY.—This rare, lethal abnormality is caused by lack of closure of the embryonic neural tube, the structure from which the brain ultimately forms. The reason for the failure of closure is not known, but the result is virtual absence of the brain or at least absence of the cerebral hemispheres. These infants usually are stillborn or die within the first week of life. Anencephaly can be diagnosed in utero by testing the amniotic fluid for the presence of high concentrations of a fetal chemical called alpha-fetoprotein.

HOLOPROSENCEPHALY.—In this developmental malformation, the brain fails to separate into symmetric hemispheres, and the result is a severely deformed single cerebrum without normal divisions. The face also reflects the failure of division, and in the most severe form of holoprosencephaly there is a single eye in the middle of the face (cyclopia). This type of malformation is incompatible with life, and such infants usually are stillborn.

CEREBRAL MALFORMATIONS

Milder forms of this anomaly exist in which the brain is only partially segmented. Facial deformities are also less severe and may include closely spaced eyes (hypotelorism), malformed nose and cleft lip and palate. Severe mental retardation is common with some types of partial holoprosencephaly.

MICROGYRIA.—This developmental disorder is characterized by malformation of the convolutions of the brain (*gyri*— see Chap. 1), resulting in very small gyri in the cerebral hemispheres. This abnormality is associated with severe mental retardation, microcephaly and seizures. There probably is no single cause of this malformation. Microgyria has been associated with intrauterine viral infections but many times a specific cause cannot be found.

HYDROCEPHALUS.—This term refers to enlargement of the fluid-filled areas inside the brain (ventricles) due to an increase in the amount of cerebrospinal fluid (CSF). The result is an infant with an enlarged head size because of increased pressure from the ventricles expanding the bones of the infant's skull. Abnormal accumulations of cerebrospinal fluid may be the result of increased production or decreased absorption. In infants with hydrocephalus, the cause usually is impairment of absorption of CSF. This may occur in one of two ways. Blockage of normal flow through the ventricular system (*noncommunicating hydrocephalus*) can occur, for example, with *aqueductal stenosis*. (The aqueduct of Sylvius is a narrow channel that connects parts of the ventricular system.) Direct blockage of reabsorption of CSF (communicating hydrocephalus) is also possible. The sites of CSF absorption are the *arachnoid villi*, small masses of cells on the surface of the brain. Arachnoid villi can be blocked by scarring, which may occur after meningitis or encephalitis or after bleeding around the brain (subarachnoid hemorrhage).

Narrowing of the aqueduct of Sylvius and other forms of noncommunicating hydrocephalus can also result from scar formation after meningitis and encephalitis and from congenital malformations. A rapid increase in size of an infant's head out of proportion to normal growth for that age suggests the

44 Structural Diseases of the Nervous System

possibility of hydrocephalus. Computerized tomography of the head is the diagnostic tool of choice to demonstrate enlarged ventricles (Fig. 5–1). Treatment consists of a shunt procedure, in which one end of a small tube is placed into a ventricle inside the brain; the tube is brought out through a small hole in the skull and placed under the skin from the head to the abdomen. The other end of the tube empties into a space inside the abdomen (ventriculoperitoneal shunt). Excess fluid can in this way drain from the ventricles and be reabsorbed inside the peritoneal cavity by the blood stream, thus preventing overaccumulation of fluid inside the brain. Fluid can be shunted to other areas of the body as well by placing the tube into the right atrium of the heart (ventriculoatrial shunt) or into the pleural space of the chest (ventriculopleural shunt).

Shunt procedures are quite effective in treating hydrocephalus. Complications of this type of surgery can include infections (which may lead to meningitis, since one end of the tube is inside the brain) and blockage of the tubing, which may lead to symptoms of acute hydrocephalus (headache, vomiting, irritability, lethargy) because the excess fluid cannot be removed adequately.

Fig. 5–1.—CT scan of patient with enlarged ventricles (hydrocephalus) is shown in right photo. Comparison of ventricular size should be made with normal CT scan at left. Arrows point to ventricles in both scans.

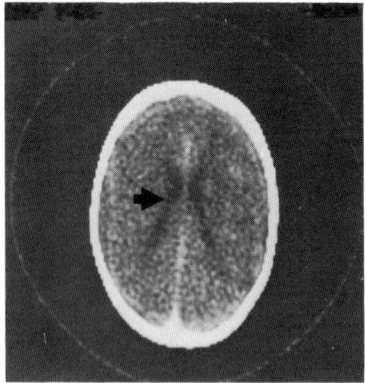
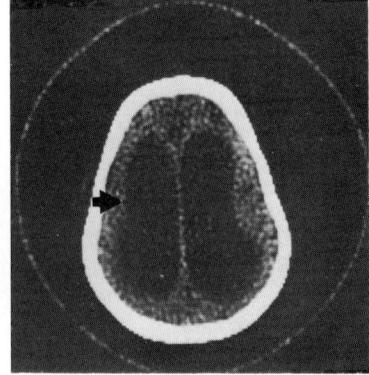

CEREBRAL MALFORMATIONS

There are other causes of large heads (macrocephaly) besides hydrocephalus. Macrocephaly may be familial and totally benign, with no identifiable abnormalities. On the other hand, certain metabolic diseases of the nervous system, for example, Tay-Sachs, are accompanied by a large head size, and the *neurocutaneous syndromes* (especially neurofibromatosis) may also have macrocephaly as a feature.

MICROCEPHALY.—This term means "small head." If a child's head is smaller than normal (more than 2 standard deviations below the mean head circumference for age) he is by definition microcephalic. Abnormally small head size indicates impairment in brain growth and usually, although *not invariably*, is associated with intellectual impairment.

Microcephaly may be primary or secondary. The primary form is inherited in an autosomal recessive fashion (see Chap. 6). These children have a receding forehead and large-appearing face and ears in contrast to the small head. They usually are mentally retarded and may have mild spasticity.

Chromosomal abnormalities and intrauterine infections may produce significant damage to the developing nervous system, and microcephaly can be an accompanying feature of these problems.

Damage to the brain in the perinatal period can produce an arrest in brain growth and secondary microcephaly. Lack of oxygen, infections of the nervous system and metabolic disorders can result in microcephaly, usually accompanied by other neurologic problems, such as seizures, spasticity and psychomotor retardation.

PORENCEPHALY.—This disorder is marked by abnormal cavities within the brain substance, which usually communicate with but are not a normal part of the ventricles. These cavities are produced by destruction of part of the brain, usually as a result of an intrauterine stroke or *cerebral infarction*. The dead tissue becomes liquefied, the liquid eventually becomes absorbed and a hole is left (Fig. 5–2).

Clinical manifestations of porencephaly depend on the area of the brain that has been damaged. Hemiparesis and seizures are common sequelae.

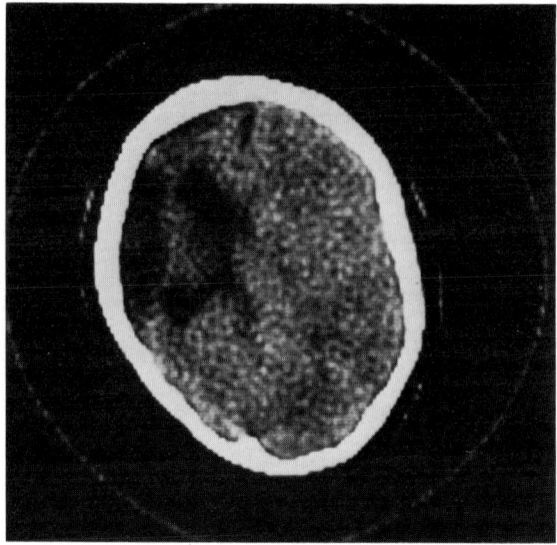

Fig. 5–2.—CT scan of a 15-year-old patient with porencephaly. Note asymmetry of skull due to underlying hemiatrophy of brain.

CEREBELLAR MALFORMATIONS

CEREBELLAR AGENESIS.—Part or all of the cerebellum may fail to form during embryonic development. Complete absence or agenesis of the cerebellum is rare, but moderate degrees of underdevelopment are common. Many people with cerebellar agenesis have no demonstrable neurologic abnormalities.

DANDY-WALKER SYNDROME.—This entity is characterized anatomically by cystic dilatation of the fourth ventricle, which is adjacent to the cerebellum, and by obstructive hydrocephalus. The cerebellum is malformed and other brain anomalies may be associated as well; these include microgyria, aqueductal stenosis and syringomyelia (see below).

Clinically, children with Dandy-Walker syndrome may exhibit a wide range of neurologic abnormalities. Most prominent are delayed motor development, ataxia, poor coordination and jerky movements of the eyes (nystagmus). The back of the head appears much more prominent than normal on examination. In later childhood, hydrocephalus may worsen and symptoms of irritability, headaches and vomiting can develop.

Treatment consists of a neurosurgical procedure in which a shunt tube is placed within the cyst to drain fluid and to relieve pressure.

ARNOLD-CHIARI MALFORMATION.—In this anomaly there is a developmental abnormality of the cerebellum and brainstem that causes these structures to be displaced downward into the spinal canal. Since the spinal canal is narrow, symptoms result from compression of the displaced structures. Four types of Arnold-Chiari malformations have been described, based on the degree of displacement of cerebellum and brainstem.

Symptoms depend on the degree of severity of the malformation. In milder forms, the child may be asymptomatic for many years or demonstrate only mild signs of cerebellar dysfunction, such as ataxia and nystagmus. In more severe forms, hydrocephalus (from blockage of normal cerebrospinal fluid flow) is an early feature (Fig. 5–3). Treatment consists of a

Fig. 5–3.—CT scan of an 18-year-old patient with Arnold-Chiari malformation and associated hydrocephalus. There is generalized dilatation throughout the ventricular system.

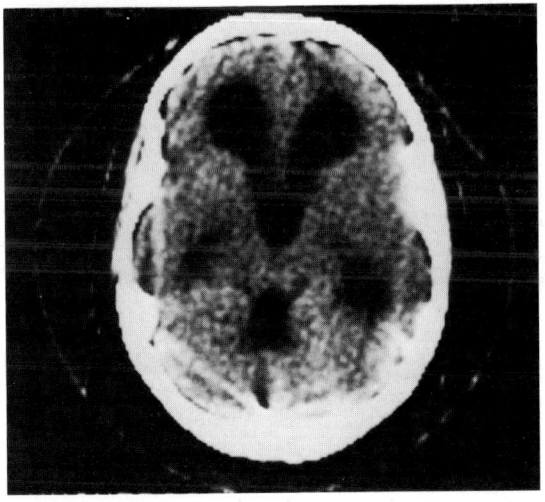

shunt procedure to relieve hydrocephalus and decompression of the cerebellum and brainstem by removal of overlying bone and membranous coverings.

CRANIOSYNOSTOSIS

Premature closure of one or more *sutures* (gaps between bones of the infant's skull) is called craniosynostosis. The cause of this anomaly is not known. The sutures may be closed at birth or may fuse in the first few months of life. Abnormalities in the shape of the head result from premature closure of sutures. The brains of patients with craniosynostosis are normal and continue to grow in every direction they can despite the closed sutures. This restricted direction of growth produces abnormal head shapes.

SCAPHOCEPHALY.—This is the term applied to an elongated head that results from premature closure of the sagittal suture. These children usually have normal neurologic function but have a cosmetic defect due to the odd shape of the head.

ACROCEPHALY.—This refers to a foreshortened head due to premature closure of the coronal sutures.

OXYCEPHALY ("TOWER HEAD").—This results from closure of both coronal and sagittal sutures. The only direction in which the brain can grow is upward, and the head shape is tall and narrow. Increased intracranial pressure may result from this type of bony fusion.

PLAGIOCEPHALY.—When a suture closes on only one side of the head, a marked asymmetry in head shape results. This is called plagiocephaly and is due to unilateral closure of a coronal suture.

Treatment of craniosynostosis is based on two considerations: functional impairment in brain growth by the closed bones and cosmetic problems. Treatment consists of surgically recreating a suture between two bones to permit continued symmetric head growth. Surgery should be performed in the first year of life, since most of the brain's growth takes place during that time.

SPINAL CORD ANOMALIES AND VERTEBRAL DEFECTS

SPINA BIFIDA. — This refers to incomplete closure of one or more vertebrae or bones of the spinal column (Fig. 5-4). If only a bony defect is present, it is called *spina bifida occulta* (Fig. 5-5). A bifid spine may occur anywhere along the spinal column from top (cervical spine) to bottom (lumbosacral spine). There may be no detectable neurologic deficit from this anomaly in development and many cases are asymptomatic. When such a vertebral defect is present there may be a small tuft of hair or a dimple in the skin of the spine overlying the defect. In some patients with bony defects of the spine, the spinal cord may be tethered at its lower end (called the *conus medullaris*), with resultant limitation of spinal cord movement as growth occurs. This may result in subtle, pro-

Fig. 5–4. — Diagram of cross-sectional view of a lumbar vertebra.

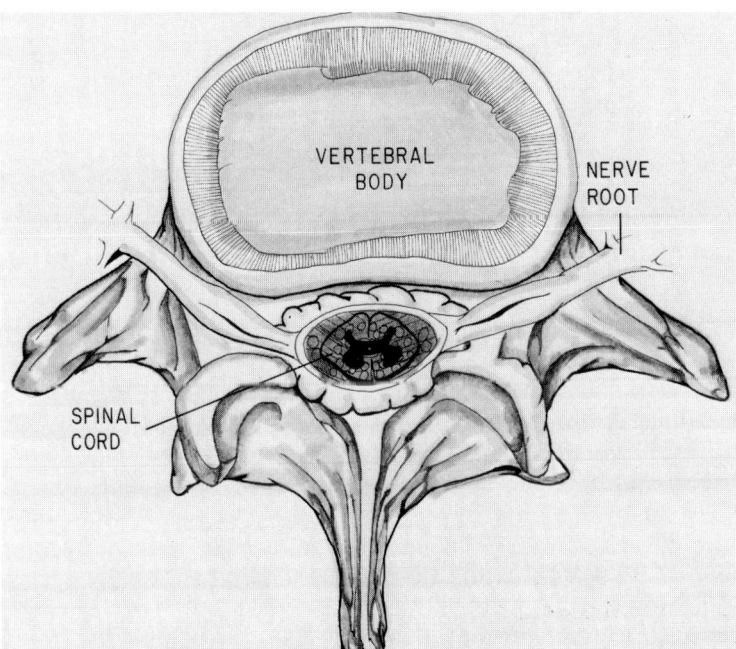

50 STRUCTURAL DISEASES OF THE NERVOUS SYSTEM

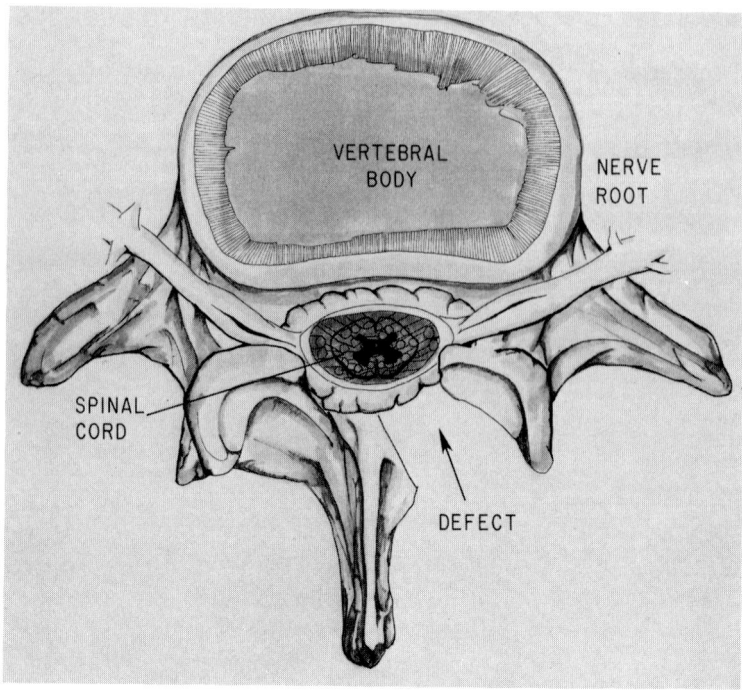

Fig. 5–5.—Diagrammatic representation of a bifid defect in a lumbar vertebra.

gressive gait or bladder disturbances as the spinal cord becomes stretched. Treatment for this condition consists of surgically freeing the lower end of the spinal cord to restore its mobility.

When a vertebra fails to close completely, some or all of the contents of the spinal canal can push through the defect and form a bulge on the back. A *meningocele* is a sac that contains the membranous coverings (meninges) of the spinal cord as well as cerebrospinal fluid (Fig. 5–6). This type of defect must be surgically corrected, since this abnormality may be accompanied by malformation of neural elements and subsequent tethering of the conus medullaris.

A more serious spinal defect is a *meningomyelocele*, a sac protruding through the bifid vertebra that contains not only

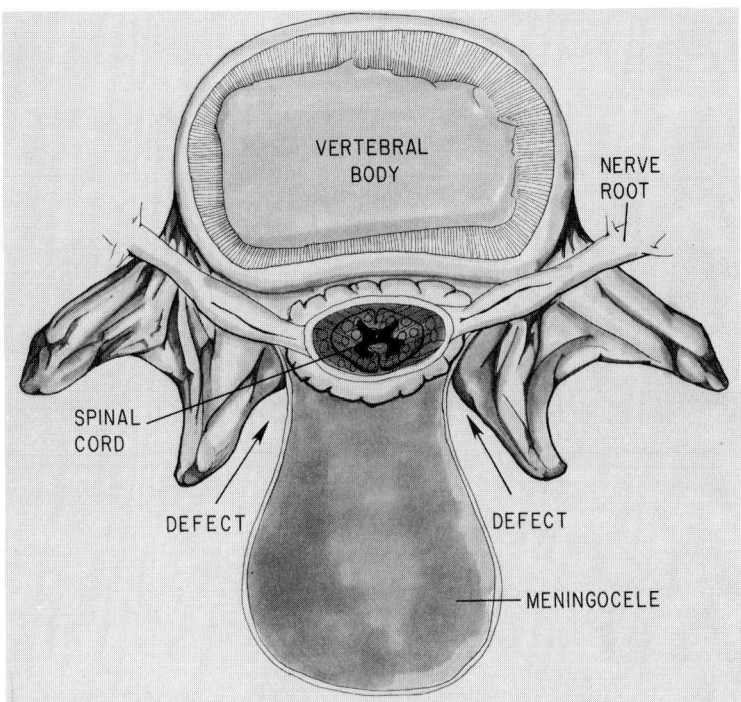

Fig. 5–6.—Diagrammatic representation of a meningocele protruding through a bifid defect in a lumbar vertebra.

meninges but part of the spinal cord as well (Fig. 5–7). This type of defect often is accompanied by paralysis of the legs, abnormalities of bladder and bowel control and foot deformities, such as clubfeet. Hydrocephalus may be an associated complication. Meningomyelocele should be corrected as soon as possible after birth, preferably within the first 24 hours of life. Early surgery may prevent further damage to the exposed spinal cord and reduce the incidence of infection.

These children frequently require long-term care by a comprehensive medical team. This includes a urologist to deal with the chronic urinary problems that these children incur due to lack of voluntary bladder control, an orthopedist to assess and treat deformities such as clubfeet and scoliosis

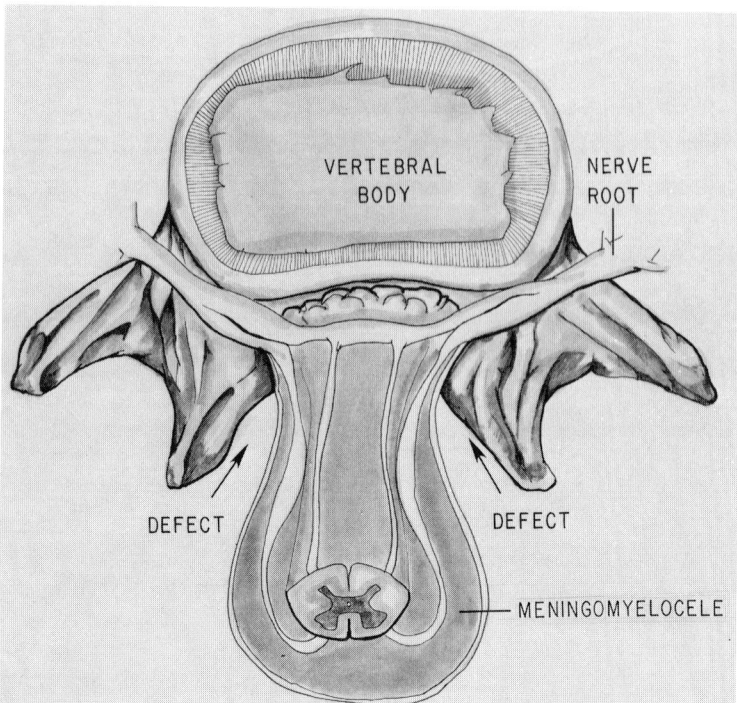

Fig. 5–7.—Bifid defect in lumbar vertebra: part of the spinal cord and its coverings protruding through the defect (meningomyelocele).

(curvature of the spine) and a rehabilitative therapist to plan and execute a physical therapy program that includes gait training, balance and coordination of lower limbs. Orthopedic devices such as braces may be necessary to correct limb deformities and to aid ambulation.

A similar defect in bony closure of the skull can occur. In this case, a portion of the brain may protrude through the defect. This is called an *encephalocele*. Treatment consists of surgical closure of the defect, but long-term neurologic deficits from brain maldevelopment may occur.

SACRAL AGENESIS.—This is another developmental defect of the spine in which the lower end of the vertebral column,

Spinal Cord Anomalies & Vertebral Defects

the *sacrum*, is absent and the lower portion of the spinal cord is malformed. Symptoms include bladder and bowel dysfunction and motor and sensory deficits in the legs. Little can be done therapeutically to correct this deformity, but gait training may have rehabilitative value. These children may never develop complete bladder and bowel control, and so may present special problems in a classroom situation.

The spina bifida defect may also be found in association with other spinal cord anomalies. *Syringomyelia* is a malformation that results in a fluid-filled cystic distortion of a portion of the spinal cord (Fig. 5–8). This abnormality may be asymptomatic during childhood, although curvature of the spine (scoliosis) and/or hydrocephalus may be accompanying features. As the child grows, the cavity (syrinx) within the spinal cord expands and eventually distorts the adjacent cord and produces symptoms that initially include decreased sensation of pain and temperature in hands and feet, and eventually produces weakness and spasticity as well. This defect cannot be repaired surgically. However, when progressive neurologic dysfunction becomes apparent, amelioration

Fig. 5–8.—Diagrammatic view of spinal cord in cross-section showing cystic distortion (syrinx).

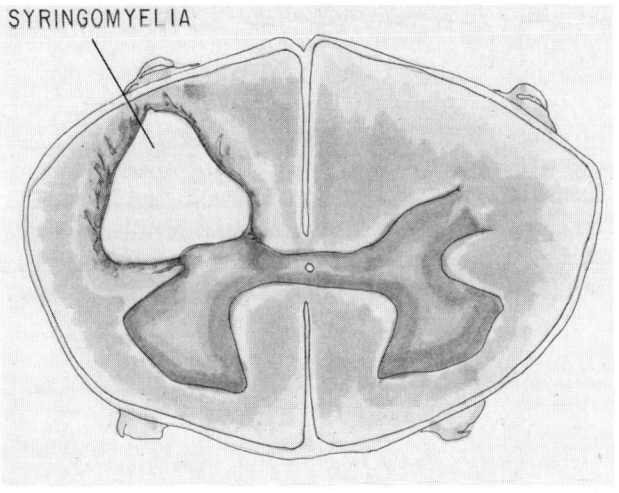

may be produced by removal of bone overlying the syrinx to decompress the enlarged spinal cord and, in some cases, by inserting a shunt tube to drain fluid from the cavity and reduce its size.

KLIPPEL-FEIL SYNDROME. — This is a developmental disorder in which two or more cervical vertebrae are fused, and in some cases there is a reduced number of vertebrae. On examination, these children have a short neck and limitation in movement of head and neck. This spinal deformity can cause compression of the spinal cord and result in progressive paraplegia in childhood. When this happens, surgical decompression of the spinal cord by removal of the overlying bone may prevent or delay further symptoms. At times, syringomyelia may be associated with this disorder.

MASS LESIONS OF THE NERVOUS SYSTEM

The brain is enclosed in a bony covering and there is little room inside the skull for any "extra" structures. Therefore, any mass that grows in or near the brain may produce symptoms in a relatively short time, primarily from compression of adjacent brain tissue.

Blood vessels course through the brain in an intricate network to supply nutrients and oxygen to all areas. Mistakes in development of cerebral blood vessels can result in a clump of enlarged arteries and veins called an *arteriovenous malformation*. Because these vessels are abnormally large, an unusually massive amount of blood flows through them, which, in turn, leads to further enlargement of the malformation. This mass may be present but asymptomatic or may produce symptoms of neurologic dysfunction, depending on the area of brain that it compresses. Progressive hemiparesis or hemisensory deficits may be seen. Irritation of underlying brain may produce a seizure disorder. At times, a *bruit,* or abnormal rushing sound, can be heard by listening to the head with a stethoscope. Arteriovenous malformations may manifest symptoms at any time during life. Occasionally an arteriovenous malformation may bleed and produce sudden onset of neurologic deficit, a type of stroke.

Diagnosis can be made by computerized tomographic scans or by a radioisotope brain scan, which outlines areas of increased blood flow. In some cases, arteriography is necessary to make the diagnosis. Arteriography is a procedure in which a special dye is injected into the blood vessels of the neck that lead into the brain. As the dye circulates through the vessels of the brain, x-rays are taken and any abnormal blood vessel malformation can be detected. When a symptomatic arteriovenous malformation is detected, in many cases total or at least partial surgical removal of the clump of vessels is possible. Prognosis depends on the number of vessels involved, the degree of damage that may have been done to underlying tissue by the malformation and the location of the malformation.

Aneurysms form another class of vascular malformation. An aneurysm is an abnormal ballooning of a segment of artery, producing a bulge in the vessel, which may act as a mass. This mass then can produce symptoms by compression or irritation of adjacent brain substance. Aneurysms can also bleed spontaneously and result in intracranial or subarachnoid hemorrhage (Fig. 5–9). The method for diagnosis of an aneurysm is essentially the same as that for an arteriovenous malformation. Treatment consists of placing a surgical clip on the neck of the aneurysm; the clip prevents blood from flowing into the aneurysm.

Tumors of the nervous system are not uncommon in children. As with tumors at any age, the underlying cause for their occurrence is not clear. In children, some tumors are associated with hereditary diseases such as tuberous sclerosis and neurofibromatosis (see Chaps. 6 and 7). Others (craniopharyngiomas, medulloblastomas) are formed from areas of maldevelopment in the brain. Whatever the cause, brain tumors can arise at any age.

Brain tumors may be benign or malignant. However, because the brain is enclosed within the bones of the skull, even a benign tumor, as it grows, will produce increased pressure inside the head. Tumors thus produce symptoms because of increased intracranial pressure or by direct compression of adjacent areas of the brain. In addition, tumors may grow within the ventricular system and obstruct normal flow of cerebrospinal fluid. Hydrocephalus then may develop.

56 STRUCTURAL DISEASES OF THE NERVOUS SYSTEM

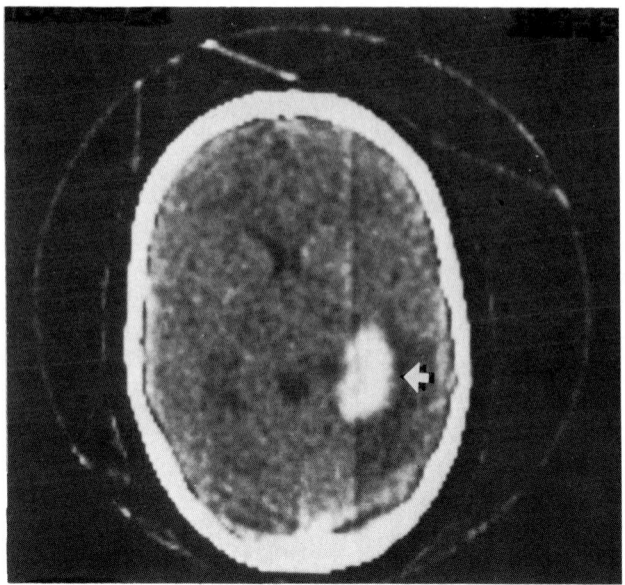

Fig. 5–9.—CT scan in a 15-year-old patient with an intracranial hemorrhage *(arrow).*

When pressure increases inside the head, the patient may develop headache and vomiting. Both of these most commonly occur in early morning. Headache pain tends to be generalized, all over the head or over the forehead, and is of little value in localizing the tumor. Double vision *(diplopia)* may also result from increased intracranial pressure because of pressure on the nerves that control eye movements.

The optic nerve in back of the eye may become swollen secondary to increased intracranial pressure. This swelling is called *papilledema* and can be detected by careful ophthalmoscopic examination of the eyes.

In infants, the bones of the skull are not yet fused and can be pushed outward by increased pressure inside the head. A rapid growth in head circumference thus may be an accompanying feature of brain tumors in infants.

When tumors compress adjacent brain tissue, they can produce symptoms of brain *irritation* (seizures) or of *destruction*

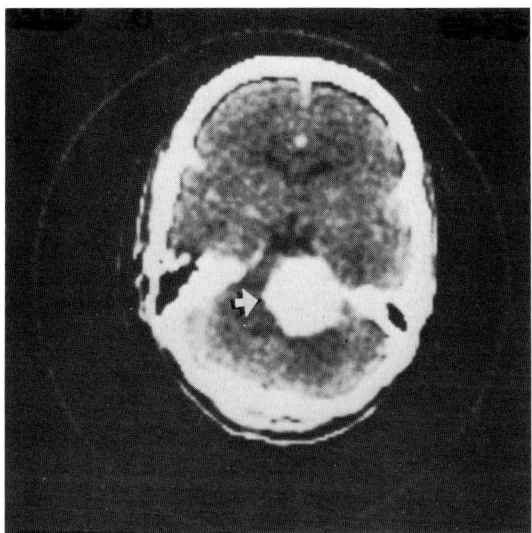

Fig. 5-10. — CT scan of a patient with a brain tumor *(arrow)*.

(for example, weakness, sensory loss). Tumors account for only a very small percentage of seizure disorders in childhood.

Sudden and abnormal increase in head size, papilledema, diplopia, early morning headache and vomiting may all suggest the possibility of a brain tumor or other mass lesion. The best noninvasive diagnostic test to detect a brain tumor is the CT scan (Fig. 5-10). Radioisotopic brain scans are also helpful in detecting the presence of mass lesions.

Treatment and prognosis depend on the type of tumor and its location. Some types of tumors are very slow-growing and well encapsulated and can be removed entirely by surgery. Others are more rapidly growing and infiltrate widely into normal brain tissue, making it impossible to remove them completely. In such cases, a combination of partial surgical removal, radiation therapy to the remainder of the tumor and the administration of anticancer drugs (chemotherapeutic agents) may be effective in eradicating the tumor, or at least in slowing its growth.

6

MENTAL RETARDATION

MENTAL RETARDATION refers to a condition in which a child has significantly subnormal intelligence. This problem is not a diagnostic entity in itself but is the result of a variety of problems, including congenital malformations of the brain, infections of the central nervous system, severe head trauma, genetic defects, chemical imbalances within the body and toxins such as lead. Some conditions that lead to mental retardation are treatable and brain damage can be prevented if the problem is diagnosed and therapy begun early. Such conditions include congenital hypothyroidism (cretinism), galactosemia and phenylketonuria. Once the brain damage has occurred, however, it usually cannot be reversed. Therefore, a search for treatable problems should be initiated immediately in any infant who appears to have a neurologic abnormality, for example, delay in development of motor milestones, or in an infant with unexplained liver enlargement or coarse or unusual facial features.

Mental testing in children generally is accomplished by the use of standardized intelligence tests. In infants and very young children it is not always possible to make a definite diagnosis of mental retardation, because cognitive skills are just developing. A developmental quotient (DQ) can be derived by dividing the child's developmental age (milestones achieved) by his chronologic age. The Denver Developmental Screening Test commonly is used to assess developmental milestones. In the preschool age group, the Stanford-Binet scale is used to assess IQ and in school-age children the Wechsler Intelligence Scale for Children (WISC) can be used. IQ tests are not infallible, of course; lack of cooperation or anxiety on the child's part can lower test results, as can uncontrollable hyperactive behavior and short attention span. However, the IQ test can be used concomitantly with evaluations of school and social performance. Developmental history and the neurologic examination are also vital in assessing the possibility of impaired mental development. When motor as well as intellectual impairment is evident, the child is said to have psychomotor retardation.

It is estimated that there is a prevalence rate of mental retardation of approximately 3% in the United States. In general, a child is considered mentally retarded if the IQ is below 70. An IQ between 50 and 70 is considered mildly retarded and such children are educable; that is, in many instances they can learn some classroom skills. These people often are capable of independent care and can be trained for vocational skills. The 30–50 range is considered moderately retarded and these children are trainable, that is, able to learn self-care skills. Below an IQ of 30 most children require custodial care and close supervision.

CAUSES OF MENTAL RETARDATION

GENETIC. — Abnormalities in chromosome patterns are responsible for some cases of mental retardation. The most common and well-known chromosome abnormality is Down's syndrome (see Chap. 7). Down's syndrome (mongolism) is caused by an extra chromosome (number 21). Mental retardation, typical facial appearance, loose, hyperextensible joints, decreased muscle tone and heart defects are among the characteristic features of Down's syndrome. Almost all children with Down's syndrome have some degree of mental retardation, but the range may vary from almost normal intelligence to severe retardation.

There are many inherited problems aside from chromosome anomalies that are associated with mental retardation. Some of these include the neurocutaneous syndromes, in which central nervous system maldevelopment is coupled with characteristic skin changes. For example, tuberous sclerosis is a neurocutaneous syndrome that is inherited in a dominant fashion; that is, if one parent has this entity, statistically

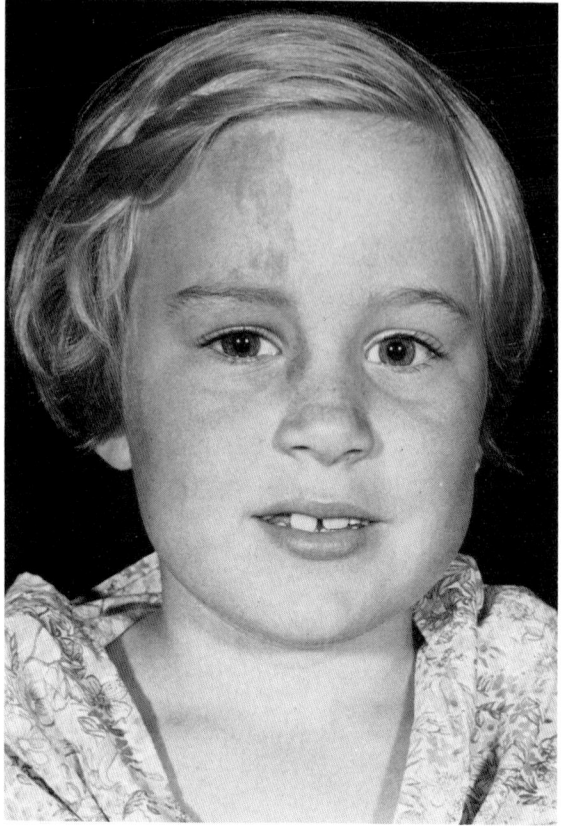

Fig. 6–1.—A 5-year-old girl with Sturge-Weber syndrome with typical port-wine nevus on forehead. This child also has glaucoma. She has normal intelligence and no intracranial calcifications.

one-half of his or her children would be affected as well. The skin manifestations of tuberous sclerosis include small areas of depigmentation, rough patches of skin (shagreen spots), a facial rash superficially resembling acne (adenoma sebaceum) and small wart-like tumors in the gums and under the fingernails (subungual fibromas). Mental retardation, seizures and central nervous system malformations are present in some, but not all, patients with tuberous sclerosis.

Sturge-Weber syndrome is another neurocutaneous syndrome that may result in intractable seizures and mental retardation. The typical skin manifestation is a "port wine" stain over the upper part of the face, usually on one side only (Fig. 6–1). People with Sturge-Weber syndrome may also have large vascular malformations inside the brain, which eventually calcify and can be detected on x-rays of the skull as a "railroad track" pattern of calcification (Fig. 6–2). These malformations are easily demonstrated by computerized tomography (CT) scan also (Fig. 6–3). When calcifications are present, patients usually have severe seizures that are difficult to control. Mental retardation is a variable occurrence in Sturge-Weber syndrome but, when present, may be quite profound.

Another complication of this disorder is glaucoma, or increased pressure within the eye; this can lead to blindness if untreated. All children with the cutaneous signs of Sturge-

Fig. 6–2.—Skull x-ray from an 18-year-old girl with Sturge-Weber syndrome showing intracranial calcifications (arrow). This patient is mildly retarded and has severe seizures.

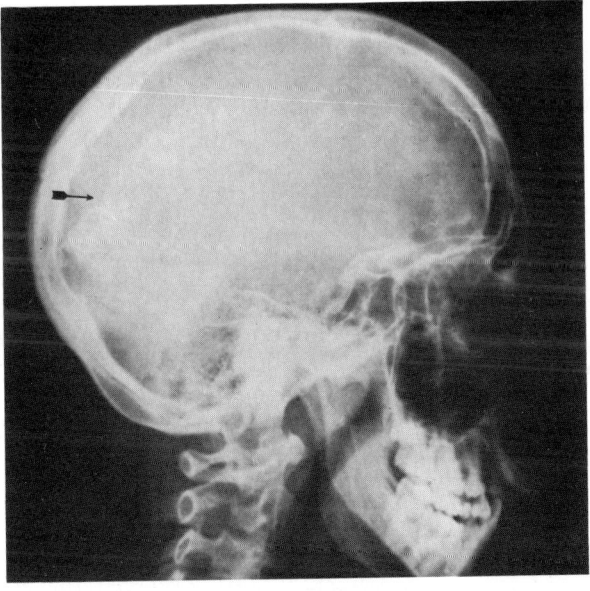

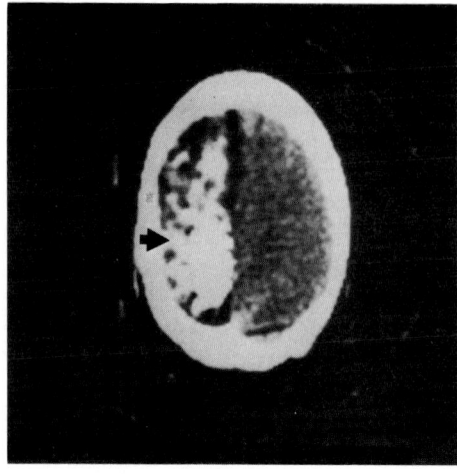

Fig. 6–3.—Computerized tomographic scan of an 18-year-old girl with Sturge-Weber syndrome demonstrating massive intracranial calcifications in the left hemisphere *(arrow)*.

Weber should be checked from early life by an ophthalmologist.

Phenylketonuria (PKU) is an inherited defect of amino acid metabolism in which the body cannot use phenylalanine properly; as a result, this substance accumulates in large quantities. Children with PKU are normal at birth, but at the age of about 6 months develop seizures, progressive loss of developmental functions and a typical type of skin rash, or eczema. Untreated, abnormal accumulation of phenylalanine eventually produces brain damage and results in mental retardation. The retardation is preventable by early diagnosis and maintenance of a special low phenylalanine diet. Since the introduction of routine screening of newborns for PKU, the neurologic consequences of this disease have been reduced greatly.

CONGENITAL.—At times, a mistake occurs during fetal development and the nervous system is malformed. When this happens, the brain usually cannot function in a normal manner, and psychomotor retardation may be the result. Examples of maldevelopment include abnormalities in configuration and size of the convolutions of the brain (polymicrogyria, pachygyria), absence of fiber tracts that normally connect the two hemispheres of the brain (agenesis of corpus callosum) and even absence of brain cortex (anencephaly).

The causes of most cases of brain maldevelopment are not known; fortunately, these abnormalities are rare. When present, there is no treatment, since the brain itself is so malformed.

INFECTIOUS. — Any infection that involves the central nervous system carries the potential danger of damage to the brain. Since the brain cells do not regenerate to any significant extent, such damage may be permanent. The complications of meningitis and encephalitis are discussed more fully in Chapter 11.

CONGENITAL INFECTIONS. — Many microorganisms can exist within the human body undetected because they produce only subtle symptoms of illness. But these same agents can be quite destructive if they invade the developing fetus. Infants born after infection *in utero* may have severe neurologic problems, including microcephaly, mental retardation, spasticity and hydrocephalus.

The infectious diseases that commonly are associated with these congenital abnormalities include cytomegalic inclusion disease, toxoplasmosis, herpesvirus, rubella and syphilis.

Congenital infection should be suspected in an infant whose weight and length are below normal, or who has early jaundice with an enlarged liver, seizures soon after birth and either a smaller than normal head due to failure of brain growth or a larger than normal head due to hydrocephalus. Toxoplasmosis and syphilis can be treated with antibiotics, and it is important to make the diagnosis early in order to prevent further damage, which could be caused by the continued presence of infection.

METABOLIC. — Many types of chemical or metabolic imbalance in the body can affect the nervous system. At times, the problem is transient and reversible with treatment. If there is a prolonged or repetitive chemical abnormality, however, damage to the nervous system may be permanent. Common chemical imbalances include hypoglycemia (low blood sugar), alterations of electrolyte (salt) concentrations in blood (for example, low sodium [hyponatremia]) and abnormal accumulation of chemicals because of a block in their utilization or breakdown (for example, PKU). Many of the metabolic abnormalities are treatable.

Hyponatremia and other electrolyte abnormalities may be found after prolonged diarrhea or vomiting, especially when accompanied by the ingestion of very dilute liquids or water, which do not adequately replace the salt lost. Water intoxication is seen most commonly when there is inappropriate secretion of pituitary antidiuretic hormone; for instance, during acute infections of the central nervous system. In water intoxication, water moves into brain cells at a rapid rate, disturbing the normal cellular equilibrium. The function of these "swollen" cells is impaired, and the patient may become drowsy or comatose. Seizures occur regularly. Damage to the nervous system may be irreversible. Treatment is aimed at correcting the fluid and electrolyte imbalance, but cautiously, since sudden shifts in any direction may be harmful. The treatment of water intoxication, as opposed to hyponatremia with dehydration, is fluid restriction.

Low blood sugar (hypoglycemia) has many causes. Since the brain uses glucose as an energy source, prolonged deficiency of this chemical can be detrimental to brain cell function. Treatment is aimed at increasing the concentration of blood sugar and preventing further episodes of hypoglycemia by appropriate dietary modifications based on the underlying cause of the hypoglycemia.

Diabetes mellitus can occur in children as well as in adults. Such patients are unable to utilize glucose adequately because of a relative lack of insulin. Glucose eventually accumulates in the blood (hyperglycemia). The blood thus becomes too concentrated (hyperosmolar state) and fluid shifts can occur. Coma and sudden increases of pressure in the brain can ensue if these shifts are severe. Residual brain damage may result from severe pressure and prolonged coma. Diabetes is a lifelong problem; as yet there is no cure. There is

Causes of Mental Retardation

treatment, however, using insulin injections and special diets to control the levels of glucose.

Reye's syndrome is an acute process seen only in children. This entity has gained much recognition in the past few years. The cause of Reye's syndrome is not known. Although it usually follows a viral illness, it does not appear to be the direct result of an infectious agent. The diagnosis is made from the history and specific laboratory examinations. Typically, the child is recovering from a viral illness when there is the sudden onset of repeated vomiting followed shortly by lethargy, coma and, at times, seizures. Laboratory studies show abnormalities in tests of liver function, prolonged blood-clotting times and hypoglycemia, especially in children under the age of 3 years. The brain becomes massively swollen, to the point where blood flow to the brain cells may be compromised.

Treatment consists of intensive supportive care, maintenance of adequate breathing, correction of chemical abnormalities in the blood and removal of excess fluid from the brain by the use of dehydrating agents, which help to decrease brain swelling.

The mortality from Reye's syndrome is significant (up to 40%) and, in survivors, permanent brain damage, including mental retardation, may result from the massive swelling and impairment of blood flow through the brain. At present there is no way to prevent Reye's syndrome, but, with earlier recognition and aggressive therapy, the mortality and other consequences of this disease are beginning to decline.

TOXINS. — Many substances are poisonous to the body, especially in large amounts. Small children explore their environment in many ways. One of the earliest is through oral contact, and many things enter the mouths of children that are not meant to be eaten. Lead poisoning can cause brain damage and mental retardation. Lead is found in old paint on walls, which can be scraped or peeled off and eaten by inquisitive children. Lead is also found in some types of pottery that may be used as eating utensils, in old pewter and in the dust around some factories; for example, those manufacturing lead pipes. All of these are potential sources for lead ingestion.

Lead poisoning may take two forms, acute and chronic. In the acute form, very large amounts of lead are ingested in a short time and the blood lead concentration is raised dramatically. The symptoms of acute lead poisoning include stomach upset, vomiting, headache, seizures and coma, with swelling of brain cells. This process can be fatal. In chronic lead poisoning, smaller amounts of lead accumulate over a longer period, and symptoms are more insidious. Irritability, hyperactivity, anemia and stomach upset may be the only signs for awhile. Eventually, seizures, mental retardation or other evidence of neurologic damage may be found.

Severe lead poisoning may result in permanent brain damage and mental retardation. A high index of suspicion should alert those who work with children to the possibility of lead poisoning in a child who shows any of the above signs, especially if the population involved is at "high risk"; for example, families living in older inner city dwellings with paint peeling off the walls.

The diagnosis of lead poisoning may be made by measuring the concentration of lead in the blood. Normally, no lead should be present; a lead level of 30 micrograms percent or greater is cause for concern. Treatment of lead poisoning consists of administering a chelating agent, which binds the lead and pulls it out of the tissues. The lead combined with the chelating agent then is excreted from the body. As with many of the disorders discussed here, early diagnosis and treatment are of paramount importance in preventing neurologic complications.

The "Fetal Alcohol Syndrome" is a disorder in which a set of characteristic abnormalities is seen in infants born to mothers who consumed large quantities of alcohol during pregnancy. Such children may have growth deficiency, microcephaly, developmental delay and mental deficiency. The damage is irreversible; treatment is a matter of prevention by educating women of childbearing age about the dangers of alcohol to the developing fetus.

TRAUMA. — Repeated or severe blows to the head may cause bleeding into and around the brain, fluid accumulation inside the head and scar formation in the brain itself. These can potentially cause permanent brain damage. It is impossible to protect a child from all accidental injuries, but one form of trauma that is all too common and is preventable is child abuse. A history of repeated episodes of broken bones, multiple fractures or unexplained or bizarre burns and bruises on the child's body should suggest the possibility of child abuse.

In the past, many people were hesitant to voice their suspicions to proper authorities for fear of parental reprisal or litigation. However, most states now have laws that protect the person reporting such suspicions. One can consult the local child welfare agency or community social service organization for details.

ENVIRONMENTAL. — Severe nutritional inadequacies deprive the body of the necessary elements for normal growth. The developing brain is particularly susceptible to nutritional deprivation. This may occur in several ways: (1) severe poverty with inability to obtain adequate food, (2) ignorance of well-balanced diet planning and bizarre "fad" diets and (3) serious mental illness in the parent, with subsequent inattentiveness to or "punishment" of the child. Prolonged and severe malnutrition may result in mental as well as growth retardation.

Care of the Mentally Retarded Child

Once a diagnosis of mental retardation has been made, it is important to place the child in an educational situation that will provide optimal stimulation. In this way, the child can achieve his maximal potential. Often, a diagnosis of mental retardation causes parents to feel that the situation is hopeless, and they do not seek special assistance. Rather, these children become overprotected and overly cared for, but are not given the stimulation needed to develop as independently as possible. This is especially the case for children in the mildly mentally retarded range, who are capable, in many instances, of independent functioning.

Stimulation should be begun early. Preschool or headstart programs often have special classes for developmentally delayed children. Retarded children who also have motor or speech handicaps sometimes can benefit from special speech and physical therapy programs. Many times, these programs can help the child to develop self-confidence, which carries over to the school programs.

Special education classes within the public school are designed to deal with the problems of mentally retarded children. Each child should be carefully evaluated and placed in a classroom that will allow him to learn at a pace at which he is capable. A child who is placed in a class that is too far above or too far below him will not be able to benefit maximally from such education.

Parental involvement is of great importance, both in the school setting and in a speech, occupational or physical therapy program. Instructors should maintain open communication with parents and, where possible, instruct parents on home programs that can help the child to develop specific skills. The ultimate developmental skills of a retarded child can be maximized by cooperative involvement of parents, teachers and health care professionals.

7

GENETIC AND METABOLIC DISORDERS

GENETICS is the study of heredity. Hereditary factors are responsible for many basic characteristics of the individual. Hair and eye color, height and skin pigmentation are determined genetically. Environmental (acquired) conditions can affect heredity, as in the malnourished child whose height is impaired because of poor nutrition. Sometimes it is difficult to separate hereditary from environmental effects in neurologic disorders. For example, epilepsy is a symptom of underlying brain dysfunction. The cause of the epilepsy may be hereditary, as in a disorder called tuberous sclerosis, or the cause may be environmental, as in post-traumatic epilepsy.

It is important to differentiate between genetic and acquired causes of disease. Treatment may be affected by the underlying cause. The ultimate outlook (prognosis) in terms of disease progression may be different in genetic and acquired defects. And, finally, patients and family may need counseling regarding the possibility of future occurrence of the same disorder in other family members. Young parents may wish to have more children and would like to know the risk of having another affected child. Therefore, a thorough knowledge of hereditary problems is necessary for genetic counseling.

A birth defect may be genetic (present because of inherited factors) or congenital. With congenital problems, the child is born with a defect because of some abnormality during intrauterine development. Certain infections (for example, syphilis, rubella) and drugs (such as alcohol) that the mother acquires or takes during pregnancy may cause abnormalities in the offspring that are obvious soon after birth. These are not hereditary, however, and the likelihood of a future pregnancy resulting in a child with similar problems is related solely to circumstances, e.g., continued presence of infection or use of alcohol by the mother.

Birth defects as a consequence of genetic abnormalities have a risk of recurrence that is dependent on the type of inheritance that the trait displays (e.g., autosomal dominant, recessive). These will be discussed below.

CHROMOSOMES AND GENES

The body is made up of systems (e.g., cardiovascular, respiratory, nervous systems) that, in turn, are composed of organs (e.g., heart, lungs, kidneys) and tissues (e.g., connective tissue). The basic element of organs and tissues is the cell. Cells are units of activity in the body. They are specialized to carry out certain functions (e.g., heart cells contract to pump blood). Each cell is composed of cytoplasm, which contains many chemicals and small substructures, and a nucleus, which contains chromosomes. Chromosomes contain the genetic information that tells each cell what its function is. This genetic information, in the form of a complex chemical called deoxyribonucleic acid (DNA), is arranged in units of information called genes.

Humans have 46 chromosomes (23 pairs) in each cell. This includes 2 sex chromosomes and 44 autosomes. Females have 2 X chromosomes whereas males have 1 X and 1 Y as sex chromosomes. A gene located on one of the X chromosomes codes for traits that are called *sex linked.* A trait carried by a gene on one of the other 44 chromosomes is an *autosomal* trait.

The 46 chromosomes are arranged in pairs. Genes on each pair of chromosomes are paired as well. Gene pairs are called *alleles.* These alleles code for the same trait but are not necessarily identical. Genes may be dominant or recessive. A dominant gene can cause the expression of its characteristic even if its paired gene is not identical. A recessive gene must be present on both chromosomes of the pair in order for its characteristic to be expressed. For example, the gene for curly hair (C) is dominant whereas the gene for straight hair (S) is recessive. Thus, if an individual has CC or CS as a gene pair he will have curly hair. Only if he has both genes for straight hair (SS) will this trait be expressed. It is possible for a recessive gene to be carried through many generations within a family before it shows up in an affected infant, since the carrier would have to mate with another carrier before the genes were able to express themselves.

Most genetic considerations are not this simple. Many traits are coded by multiple genes (for example, hair color) and the interactions become more complicated. To further complicate matters, some traits may be dominant but have *variable penetrance.* That is, although the individual has a dominant characteristic, it may not be expressed fully.

Reproductive cells (ova in females and sperm in males) contain only one-half the number of chromosomes present in other body cells. When an ovum and sperm unite to reproduce, 23 chromosomes from the mother and 23 from the father merge to form the new offspring with 46 chromosomes. A combination of these two gene populations produces the traits that will characterize the new individual. Since the female has 2 X chromosomes, the offspring must receive an X chromosome from its mother; the male has an X and a Y, so the sex of the offspring is determined by the father's chromosome contribution.

If one parent has a dominantly inherited disease there is a 50% probability that a child of this parent will have the same problem. In the case of a recessive characteristic, each parent must have at least one recessive gene (each parent then would be a carrier for the trait but would not demonstrate any evidence of it). In this situation, the probability of an offspring having the problem is 25% for each child. If only one parent carries the recessive gene there is no way in which a child can have the disease, although if the child receives one recessive gene he then will be a carrier also.

In genetic aberrations involving the sex chromosomes, most of the known gene abnormalities occur on the X chromosome and are recessive. For this reason, most X-linked disorders are seen only in males, since males have only 1 X chromosome (the other sex chromosome in males is the Y, and the X and Y chromosomes are not paired in terms of gene populations). Females have 2 X chromosomes, and the gene would have to be present on both of these in order to produce the abnormal trait. Such an occurrence would be extremely unlikely because most X-linked disorders are not compatible with a normal life, and males with such problems would not be likely to reproduce.

GENETIC DISORDERS

Many neurologic abnormalities have a genetic basis. Tay-Sachs disease is an autosomal recessive disorder that causes abnormalities in infancy. It is found primarily in people of Jewish descent. A child with Tay-Sachs disease is typically normal in the first few months of life and then begins to lose the abilities he has acquired; he no longer can roll over or sit up. These infants also have progressive impairment of vision and the onset of seizures, usually between the ages of 6 and 12 months. Death occurs by the age of 2 years in most cases. For parents with an affected child there is a 25% chance of having a subsequent child with Tay-Sachs.

Unfortunately, there is no treatment for this devastating disease, but there is a method of detecting carriers of the recessive gene by a simple blood test. If both parents are carriers and wish to have children, the fetus can be tested for the presence of the disease in the first few months of the pregnancy by a method called amniocentesis. This technique utilizes a chemical analysis to examine the cells in a small amount of amniotic fluid removed from the mother's womb. If the fetus is affected, a therapeutic abortion may be performed, if the parents wish. Most important, if the amniocentesis is normal, parents can be assured that this unborn child will not have the disease.

Another group of genetic disorders that have significant neurologic problems associated with them are the neurocutaneous syndromes. In this group are diseases with abnormalities of the central nervous system as well as of skin. The most common of these is neurofibromatosis. Neurofibromatosis is

GENETIC DISORDERS

inherited as an autosomal dominant trait with extremely variable penetrance. Thus, for example, one person may have only the skin abnormalities (darkly pigmented areas called "café au lait" spots (Fig. 7–1), fatty-appearing tumors called plexiform neuromas and superficial wart-like growths called neurofibromas whereas other members of the family may have more nervous system involvement, including mental retardation, macrocephaly (unusually large head) or seizures. Brain and spinal cord tumors may also occur more commonly in neuro-

Fig. 7–1.—A child with neurofibromatosis, demonstrating one of the typical skin manifestations of the disease, café au lait spots on abdomen *(arrow)*.

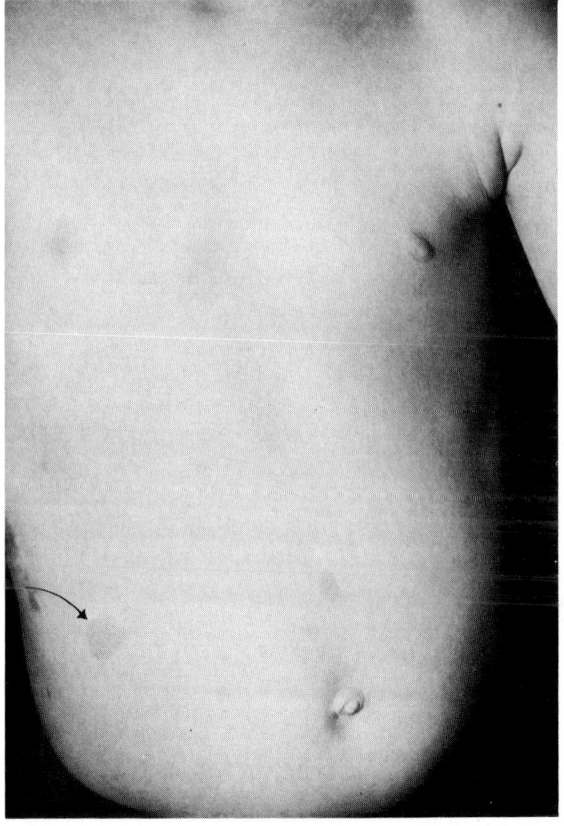

fibromatosis. These tumors usually are benign, but some eventually undergo malignant transformation. Since this disorder has dominant inheritance, if one parent has neurofibromatosis there is a 50% chance that each child will also inherit the problem.

Because of the possibility of tumor growths in such patients, it is important to know the inheritance pattern of this disorder so that the family members can be examined carefully and those with skin manifestations followed with thorough neurologic evaluations at frequent intervals so that tumors can be detected early.

Down's syndrome, which used to be called mongolism, is a disorder caused by failure of normal separation of chromosomes in the sex cells, so that the infant has an extra chromosome (trisomy 21) or an extra piece of a chromosome (15/21 translocation). When either of these occurs, the resulting offspring has the clinical features of Down's syndrome. These include characteristic facial features—mongolian slant to the eyes, round face and flat nose—hyperextensibility of the joints, decreased muscle tone, mental retardation and an increased susceptibility to leukemia, congenital heart disease and anomalies of bowel development (especially duodenal atresia, in which a part of the small bowel is abnormally narrow).

Several other chromosomal defects are known, but Down's syndrome is by far the most common.

The prognosis of genetic diseases depends on the severity of the particular disorder. A disorder such as neurofibromatosis does not necessarily have a poor prognosis, and children with neurofibromatosis who have learning disabilities or motor incoordination may derive great benefit from a program of therapy designed for their particular needs. Teachers of school-age children with neurofibromatosis can help greatly by observing the child for any change in neurologic or intellectual function, which might be the first sign of a brain tumor or of a subtle seizure disorder. It always is helpful, therefore, for the teacher, nurse or rehabilitative therapist to inquire about the nature of the neurologically impaired child's problem so as to be alert for subtle signs. Early recognition could save the child from further disabilities.

METABOLIC DISORDERS

Metabolic disorders are diseases in which a chemical imbalance in the body produces a physical abnormality. Metabolic diseases can be genetic or acquired. Many genetically caused metabolic diseases (inborn errors of metabolism) are known. These diseases result from deficient activity of an enzyme. Enzymes are specialized proteins that catalyze, or accelerate, chemical reactions in the body. These chemical reactions are necessary for the synthesis and metabolism of body proteins, fats and carbohydrates. A deficiency of a specific enzyme causes a block in the chemical reaction that that enzyme normally would catalyze, and consequently the chemical components normally used in that reaction have no place to go and accumulate in abnormally high concentrations. When this occurs, the old adage "too much of a good thing" prevails; normal, and even essential, chemicals in abnormal amounts can cause damage to body cells, with subsequent organ malfunction.

INBORN ERRORS OF AMINO ACID METABOLISM

PHENYLKETONURIA (PKU).—PKU is inherited as an autosomal recessive disorder with an incidence of 1/15,000 people in the general population. Because of an enzyme block, an amino acid, phenylalanine, accumulates in very large amounts and causes brain damage and severe mental retardation. Amino acids are small chemicals that make up proteins. Phenylalanine as well as other amino acids enter the body through the gastrointestinal tract when protein is eaten in the diet.

The presence of PKU now can be detected in the newborn by a simple blood test. Once diagnosed, patients with PKU can be treated by a special diet that has very limited amounts of phenylalanine. If the disorder is detected and treatment started in early infancy, mental retardation can be prevented and the child can develop normally.

The fact that PKU and other inherited metabolic disorders can be treated, and brain damage thus prevented, indicates the necessity for awareness of such metabolic defects by anyone dealing with infants and children.

The diet that children with PKU must follow to prevent symptoms of the disease is very restrictive. It is a hydrolysate of milk protein in which the protein is broken down into its component amino acids and then the phenylalanine removed. This formula is marketed with the trade name Lofenylac. It generally is given with small amounts of milk to provide the minimal requirements of phenylalanine. In addition to this special food, children with PKU may eat fruits and vegetables but must not eat meat, milk, cheese, nuts or other foods containing protein. Recently it has been found that in many instances this restricted diet can be liberalized, with no adverse effects, after the child reaches the age of 7 years. However, when women with PKU become pregnant, their diets again must be restricted, because high phenylalanine levels in the mothers can produce brain damage in their offspring.

MAPLE SYRUP URINE DISEASE (MSUD).—This disorder of amino acid metabolism was first described in 1954. It has an autosomal recessive inheritance pattern. The metabolic defect is a block in the normal breakdown of the three branched chain amino acids—leucine, isoleucine and valine—resulting in excessive accumulation in serum and spinal fluid of partially metabolized forms of these amino acids called ketoacids. Children with maple syrup urine disease appear normal at birth but in early infancy exhibit signs of spasticity, respiratory problems and rapid neurologic deterioration. The urine of these infants contains high concentrations of the ketoacids and has a peculiarly sweet, maple syrup odor. Diagnosis can be made by noting the peculiar odor of the urine and by analyzing the urine for ketoacids. Diagnosis can also be made in utero by chemical analysis of cells cultured from the amniotic fluid obtained by amniocentesis. Treatment is available for children with MSUD in the form of a very restricted special diet that contains minimal amounts of the amino acids leucine, isoleucine and valine. The diet must be begun very early in infancy, before irreversible neurologic damage has occurred.

HOMOCYSTINURIA.—This is the second most common inborn error of amino acid metabolism (PKU is the most common). This disorder is transmitted as an autosomal recessive problem associated with a block in the normal breakdown pathway of the sulfur-containing amino acid methionine. Infants with homocystinuria usually appear normal at birth. Symptoms may begin at about 6 months of age with seizures and slowing of development. Recurrent strokes are the hallmark of the disease. Dislocation of the lenses of the eyes (ectopia lentis) is also characteristic of homocystinuria and usually is seen after about 18 months of age.

As these children get older, they usually are mentally retarded and may have complex neurologic problems, such as hemiplegia and pseudobulbar palsy secondary to recurrent strokes.

Diagnosis can be made by testing the blood for elevated concentrations of methionine and homocystine and the urine for increased quantities of homocystine. Treatment based on restricting dietary intake of methionine and administering large amounts of vitamin B_{12} and folic acid has led to improvement in the biochemical balance in patients, but lasting improvement in neurologic status has yet to be demonstrated.

UREA CYCLE DEFECTS

Ammonia is a chemical that is produced by the body during normal breakdown of proteins and amino acids. However, ammonia itself is toxic to cells, and in order to prevent accumulation of this substance, the body quickly converts any ammonia produced to urea, which then is excreted in the urine. The series of chemical reactions by which ammonia is detoxified is collectively called the urea cycle. Five enzymes are involved in the normal function of the urea cycle. If any one of them is deficient, the cycle cannot function normally, and ammonia accumulates.

Several inborn errors of urea cycle metabolism are known. They vary in severity, but a typical patient presents in the first few days of life with repeated seizures and coma after feedings have begun (milk contains proteins and ammonia accumulates as the result of protein breakdown). In milder forms, a diet virtually devoid of protein may alleviate the symptoms, but in severe forms of the urea cycle defects, the course is rapidly progressive and fatal in a matter of days to weeks.

Diagnosis can be made by measuring the concentration of ammonia in the blood. The possibility of a urea cycle defect should be considered in any infant who develops unexplained and intractable seizures and coma in the first few days of life, or in a child who has repeated, unexplained episodes of vomiting and lethargy or coma.

ORGANIC ACID DISORDERS

Organic acids are small compounds involved in intermediate steps in metabolism. Several disorders are recognized as being the result of accumulation of organic acids because of a block in their normal metabolism.

ISOVALERIC ACIDEMIA. — This is an inborn metabolic error caused by a block in the breakdown of the amino acid leucine, with a resultant increase in concentrations of the organic acid isovaleric acid in blood. These children have a peculiar odor described as reminiscent of "sweaty feet." Symptoms include intermittent vomiting, lethargy and, at times, coma. Restriction of dietary leucine intake can help to prevent such episodes.

PROPIONIC ACIDEMIA (KETOTIC HYPERGLYCINEMIA). — This is another organic acid disorder, characterized by intermittent vomiting and lethargy, that may lead to psychomotor retardation. Symptoms can be precipitated by high dietary intake of protein.

DISORDERS OF CARBOHYDRATE METABOLISM

Numerous types of sugars are utilized by the body for normal function. Disorders of carbohydrate metabolism result in abnormalities related to the usual area of utilization of the particular sugar involved. Galactosemia is an autosomal recessive disorder in which there is a block in the body's ability to metabolize galactose. This is a simple sugar formed when

Disorders of Carbohydrate Metabolism

lactose, a disaccharide found in milk, is broken down (lactose→galactose +glucose).

Children with classic galactosemia may be normal at birth, but in the first few weeks of life develop jaundice, vomiting, diarrhea and failure to gain weight. Enlargements of liver and spleen are prominent features. Cataracts develop and neurologic deterioration, including hypotonia and loss of reflexes, becomes evident. Untreated, the disease may progress to mental retardation, cirrhosis of the liver and blindness due to cataracts.

The diagnosis can be made by finding galactose in the urine and then by documenting decreased activity of the enzyme galactose-phosphate uridyl transferase in red blood cells. Early treatment with a low galactose diet and exclusion of milk and milk products from the diet can prevent progression of symptoms and allow these children to function normally.

Pompe's disease (glycogen storage disease type II).—Glycogen is a large molecule that is made up of sugars and is a means of storing sugar in the body until needed. Glycogen storage diseases are a group of disorders in which an enzyme defect prevents normal breakdown of glycogen and results in abnormal accumulation of this compound. In Pompe's disease, glycogen accumulates in muscle, heart, liver and nervous system.

Pompe's disease usually becomes manifest in the first few months of life because of progressive muscle weakness, decreased muscle tone and enlargement of the heart. Weakness becomes severe over a few months and death occurs by about 1 year of age and usually is secondary to infection. There is no effective treatment for Pompe's disease.

Mucopolysaccharidoses.—In this group of disorders there is an abnormal accumulation in virtually every tissue in the body of complex sugar molecules called mucopolysaccharides. This accumulation produces widespread dysfunction. Hurler's syndrome (gargoylism) is one form of mucopolysaccharidosis that has an autosomal recessive inheritance. Children with Hurler's syndrome usually are normal at birth but over the first year or two of life develop very coarse facial

TABLE 7–1.—CLASSIFICATION OF THE MUCOPOLYSACCHARIDOSES

NAME	INHERITANCE	INTELLECTUAL IMPAIRMENT	BONY DEFORMITIES	CLOUDY CORNEAS	SHORT STATURE
Hurler	Autosomal recessive	Severe	Severe	Yes	Yes
Hunter	X-linked recessive	Moderate	Severe	No	Yes
Sanfilippo	Autosomal recessive	Severe	Minor	No	Mild
Morquio	Autosomal recessive	Variable	Severe	Late in course	Yes
Scheie	Autosomal recessive	None	Minor	Yes	Mild
Maroteaux-Lamy	Autosomal recessive	None	Severe	Yes	Yes

features and bony deformities (including kyphosis or humpback). Liver and spleen are enlarged and the heart valves are abnormal. These children become progressively more intellectually impaired. Some patients have hearing defects as well. Death occurs before the age of 20 and usually is due to either pneumonia or heart disease. Diagnosis is made by identifying abnormal mucopolysaccharides in the urine. There is no treatment for the mucopolysaccharidoses.

Other forms of mucopolysaccharide disorders are listed in Table 7–1.

INBORN ERRORS OF LIPID METABOLISM

Brain tissue is composed of a high proportion of fat-like chemicals called lipids. The lipidoses are hereditary disorders of lipid metabolism in which an excessive accumulation of certain brain lipids occurs. One subgroup of the lipidoses are the gangliosidoses, in which a type of lipid known as a ganglioside accumulates in the central nervous system. Tay-Sachs disease is the best known of the gangliosidoses. It now is known that the metabolic defect that produces this gangliosidosis is a deficiency in an enzyme, hexosaminidase A. Diagnosis can be made by the typical features of the disease and by measuring the activity of hexosaminidase A in the patient's blood. In Tay-Sachs disease, this activity is reduced tremendously as compared to normal. There is no treatment for this devastating disease (see earlier discussion).

Other forms of gangliosidoses exist and are differentiated by specific enzyme defects, but, in general, all of them have neurologic impairment as part of the disease and most are fatal in childhood.

Another autosomal recessive disorder of lipid metabolism is Neimann-Pick disease, which is caused by a deficiency of the enzyme sphingomyelinase. Symptoms usually begin between 3 and 9 months of age with enlargement of the liver and spleen, progressive intellectual and motor deterioration and, at times, seizures. Progression is relatively rapid and these children usually die by the age of 2 years.

Gaucher's disease is another autosomal recessive form of lipidosis that produces similar abnormalities of the central nervous system.

OTHER METABOLIC DEFECTS

LESCH-NYHAN SYNDROME.—This disorder is an X-linked recessive abnormality of purine metabolism that produces spasticity and movement disorders beginning in early childhood. The hallmark of the disease is self-mutilation, which often is quite severe and necessitates the patient being placed in restraints for his own protection.

The diagnosis can be made by the typical clinical features of the illness as well as elevations of blood levels of uric acid. The confirmatory test is based on enzymatic analysis of the blood. Antenatal diagnosis of this disease can be made.

At present there is no effective treatment for the neurologic abnormalities seen in this disorder.

HYPOTHYROIDISM. — This is a condition in which the thyroid gland is not able to produce enough thyroid hormone to meet the body's demands. Lack of thyroid hormone in infants can cause severe damage to the nervous system. The resultant infant is called a cretin: a child severely mentally retarded because of hypothyroidism before or soon after birth. Congenital hypothyroidism does occur, sometimes as a result of an autosomal recessive inheritance. Some children are born with severe neurologic impairment from birth. Unfortunately, there is little that can be done to reverse the impairment. However, some hypothyroid infants are normal at birth, and a screening blood test will detect the abnormality at this stage. If such children are detected early and treated with thyroid hormone replacement, their neurologic development may be normal.

Hypothyroidism can develop at any age. In children there is a nonhereditary, acquired type of hypothyroidism that results from an inflammation of the thyroid gland, Hashimoto's thyroiditis. This condition can have a very subtle onset, with easy fatigability, weight gain or mild muscle weakness as the only symptom. Again, awareness on the part of the professionals dealing with children can provide early detection and treatment for these patients before more serious consequences occur.

DIABETES MELLITUS. — This is a metabolic disorder in which symptoms arise because of a relative lack of insulin. Insulin is a chemical that is necessary for the utilization of sugar for the body's energy supply. In diabetes, sugar accumulates in abnormally high concentrations in the blood, causing a chemical imbalance, which may lead to coma, seizures and even death. Treatment is directed toward replacing the necessary insulin supply by daily injections and, in some cases, by

Other Metabolic Defects   83

restriction of sugar in the diet. Diabetes can occur at any age, and once it develops, requires lifelong medical attention. Children with diabetes present special problems for several reasons. First of all, and understandably, a daily injection is unpleasant and the child may rebel against these "shots." Second, dietary restrictions are especially difficult for impressionable children who want to eat what everyone else eats, and who have strong likes and dislikes with regard to food. Thus, the management of a juvenile diabetic can be a continual battle. It requires the combined support and assistance of all professionals involved with that child's educational and medical program. Poorly controlled diabetes can result in, among other things, seizures, coma and damage to nerves, which can, in turn, cause pain or weakness, especially of the legs. Therefore, it is imperative that diabetic children be well controlled medically while at the same time leading as normal and full a life as possible.

It is obvious that this chapter has covered only a very small sample of the many genetic and metabolic disorders that can produce neurologic symptoms. The general principles outlined in describing these disorders can be applied to a wide variety of neurologic problems. To summarize, these principles include the following: (1) Find out what the child has and what long-term outlook can be expected (improvement, stable problem or progressive deterioration). (2) Learn as much as possible about that particular disorder. This information can be obtained from a physician if the child's parents cannot provide sufficient explanations. (3) Be observant for any subtle signs of deterioration in attentiveness or performance, and notify parents or physician regarding such changes. Sometimes it is helpful to contact the child's physician early and ask if there are particular types of changes for which you should be especially alert.

Finally, it is important to remember that the health care professional can play a significant role even when the outlook for a particular child is grim. Physical therapy, for example, may provide supportive treatment to a severely brain-damaged child simply by preventing painful tightening of muscles and joints (contractures). It may succeed in helping make the child's life more pleasant and free from pain, and in this way help the child's family as well. And in the case of the child with an illness that requires careful management, early detection of problems can prevent serious complications and, at times, be lifesaving.

8

DEGENERATIVE DISEASES OF THE NERVOUS SYSTEM

ALTHOUGH medical science has made enormous breakthroughs in the recognition and treatment of disease in the twentieth century, there still are many diseases that are as yet largely untreatable. One such group is that of heredodegenerative diseases of the nervous system. These disorders, many of them hereditary, produce progressively severe deterioration of the brain, ultimately leading to death in most cases. Many research groups are working actively to learn more about these diseases in hopes of developing effective treatments.

Degenerative central nervous system disorders can be divided into four general groups, based on the part of the brain that is primarily affected: gray matter diseases, white matter diseases, basal ganglia disorders, cerebellar and spinal cord disorders.

The gray matter of the brain consists primarily of neuronal cell bodies. Damage to these cells produces dementia, or loss of intellectual function, and seizures. Brain white matter contains primarily axons and supportive elements. Damage to this part of the brain is likely to produce spasticity. The basal ganglia are paired subcortical structures whose function is involved with normal movement. Smooth coordination of muscle movement and maintenance of muscle tone are among the chief functions of the cerebellum.

DEGENERATIVE DISEASES INVOLVING GRAY MATTER

Alpers' syndrome (progressive poliodystrophy) is a disorder that involves selective degeneration of gray matter. Onset of symptoms usually is prior to 6 years of age, with seizures, especially myoclonic, intellectual deterioration and spasticity. These children usually die by 10 years of age and there is no known means to alter the course of the disease.

Infantile neuroaxonal dystrophy affects both gray and white matter in the brain. Symptoms usually begin prior to 1 year of age in a previously normal infant. Initial and progressive problems include spasticity, weakness, dementia, blindness and nystagmus (jerky movements of the eyes). Some children with this disease develop seizures as well. The course is somewhat protracted over 8–10 years before death.

Menkes' kinky hair syndrome (trichopoliodystrophy) is an interesting X-linked recessive disorder in which symptoms occur because of the inability of the body to effectively absorb copper. Children with this disease develop seizures, spasticity and poor weight gain within the first few months of life, with progressive mental deterioration. The hallmark of this disease is peculiarly twisted and brittle hair, which results from copper deficiency. Children with kinky hair syndrome die by the age of 2 years. Although a defect in copper metabolism is known to be the cause, as yet no effective means has been devised to remedy the problem. Administration of copper to patients has not resulted in lasting beneficial results. Studies are actively being pursued to find a way of altering the outcome of this disease.

Subacute sclerosing panencephalitis (SSPE) is a rare degenerative disease in which a slow deterioration of the brain is caused by an altered measles virus. This disease typically manifests itself between the ages of 5 and 10 years with myoclonic seizures, progressive mental deterioration and loss of speech. The usual course of the disease is about 2 years from initial symptoms to death. A new experimental drug, isoprinozine, currently is being used to treat SSPE patients. Preliminary results in a small number of patients have been promising.

Subacute necrotizing encephalomyelopathy (Leigh's disease) is a poorly understood autosomal recessive disorder that may become apparent anytime in the first few years of life, with weakness of eye muscles, swallowing difficulties, ataxia or instability of gait, seizures, nystagmus and mental deterioration. The underlying metabolic abnormality is thought to be an abnormality in pyruvate oxidation that leads to lactic acidemia. Treatment with high doses of thiamine is a controversial mode of therapy that has been tried with little success to date.

DISEASES AFFECTING PRIMARILY WHITE MATTER

Metachromatic leukodystrophy is an autosomal recessive degenerative disease produced by an abnormality of lipid metabolism in the brain. It is due to a deficiency of an enzyme, aryl sulfatase A. Onset of symptoms usually is in the second or third year of life, with ataxia, impairment of speech, spasticity, tremors and athetoid movements of the extremities. A peripheral neuropathy usually is present as well, and deep tendon reflexes are decreased or absent. Intellectual deterioration occurs gradually. There is unrelenting progression to death within 6 months to 4 years after symptoms appear in most patients. Diagnosis is made by the biochemical determination of the activity of aryl sulfatase A in white blood cells or cultured fibroblasts. There is no treatment for this disorder.

Globoid cell leukodystrophy (Krabbe's disease) is another disorder that comes about because of an abnormality in lipid metabolism. In these patients there is a deficiency of the enzyme galactocerebrosidase, and demonstration of decreased activity of this enzyme in white blood cells or skin fibroblasts helps to make the diagnosis. Symptoms usually begin at 4–6 months of age with irritability and increasing spasticity. Blindness develops and deep tendon reflexes are diminished. This disease usually is fatal by 1–2 years of age, and as yet there is no effective means of preventing disease progression.

Adrenoleukodystrophy is an X-linked recessive disorder, seen only in males, in which progressive spasticity, visual and mental deterioration beginning between the ages of 5 and 10 years are coupled with malfunction of the adrenal glands, with resultant increase in skin coloration. Adrenoleukodystrophy has a rapid course of deterioration and death in 1–2 years. No treatment is available at present.

DEGENERATIVE DISEASES OF THE BASAL GANGLIA

Huntington's chorea is an autosomal dominant disorder seen generally in adults, but onset can be in childhood and has been reported as early as 4 years of age. Symptoms of juvenile Huntington's disease include rigidity, dementia and seizures. The course is variable and slowly progressive, and there is no effective treatment, although haloperidol can decrease the abnormal movements for several years in some patients.

Wilson's disease is an autosomal recessive disorder that is caused by a defect in copper metabolism. Unlike the kinky hair syndrome, however, patients with Wilson's disease accumulate too much copper in vital organs such as liver and brain. Onset can be in children or young adults, and initial symptoms may be from liver disease or nervous system abnormalities. Neurologic problems include movement disorders (primarily dystonia), dementia and personality problems. If diagnosed early, Wilson's disease can be effectively treated by the oral administration of penicillamine, a chelating agent that binds copper and pulls it out of tissues. Copper and penicillamine then are excreted from the body in the urine.

Dystonia musculorum deformans exists in two hereditary forms. The autosomal dominant form has been found in patients with varied ethnic backgrounds. Onset of symptoms is variable and the initial symptoms may begin in children, adolescents or young adults. Involuntary writhing movements and abnormal postures are the primary abnormalities. These symptoms increase with stress initially, but as the disease progresses, voluntary movements become impossible and the patient remains fixed in very abnormal postures.

The only form of treatment that has met with some success is surgical ablation of an area of the brain, the ventrolateral nucleus of the thalamus. About three-fourths of patients with dystonia musculorum deformans achieve significant relief from symptoms with this procedure, but some patients require repeated operations before symptoms abate significantly.

SPINOCEREBELLAR DEGENERATIONS

This group of diseases involves slow loss of cells in the cerebellum, spinal cord and brainstem. Many tend to be familial, with variable inheritance patterns, and symptoms may vary widely from one family to another. Friedreich's ataxia is the most common of the spinocerebellar degenerations and is characterized by progressive ataxia, loss of coordination, speech difficulties, foot and spine deformities, impaired vibration and position senses, absence of deep tendon reflexes, atrophy of distal muscles of hands and feet and cardiac abnormalities (myocarditis). Symptoms usually begin between 10 and 20 years of age and progress slowly over many years. In advanced cases, patients are bedridden, and death usually is caused by infection or heart disease. Although no effective means is available to prevent disease progression, youngsters with Friedreich's ataxia should be kept mobile as long as possible with the help of a physical therapy program.

Charcot-Marie-Tooth disease (peroneal muscular atrophy) is a familial degenerative process that demonstrates nearly every type of inheritance pattern. Symptoms usually begin between 5 and 20 years, with weakness and atrophy of distal leg muscles followed by weakness of hand muscles. Foot deformities eventually develop (either clubfoot or pes cavus deformity). Vibratory and position senses are impaired in the feet and hands. Progression is slow over many years, and a well-planned physical therapy program can help to keep these patients active for long periods.

Many other heredodegenerative diseases affecting specific parts of the nervous system have been described. Most of them are quite rare.

9

CEREBRAL PALSY

IT IS IMPOSSIBLE to give a precise definition of cerebral palsy, because there is no specific cause or single entity to which one can refer as "cerebral palsy." The term is a descriptive one that signifies a nonprogressive impairment in brain function occurring in the prenatal, natal (birth) or early postnatal period that produces a motor deficit. Children with such a problem will not get worse over the years and this fact is quite important to remember in terms of parental counseling and planning rehabilitative programs. There is no single underlying cause of cerebral palsy. In most cases there is a history of transient anoxia (lack of oxygen to the brain) or a problem in the perinatal period, such as prematurity, prolonged labor or precipitous delivery.

The range of motor dysfunction in cerebral palsy is extremely large, varying from essentially normal ability, except for "clumsiness," to severe disability, with spasticity and weakness of all four extremities.

When the motor system is impaired secondary to diffuse brain damage there is interference with normal movement and also with maintenance of posture, balance and coordination. Motor development proceeds in a very disorganized manner and a child may attempt to circumvent his handicap by adopting different habits for walking and balance. For instance, a child with spasticity of the legs may be able to walk, but does so by walking on his toes. His gait may have a very wide base, that is, his feet are spread apart when walking, in order to maintain balance. He may achieve the goal of walking, but in a very abnormal way.

Primitive reflexes (for example, tonic neck reflex—see Chap. 1) often are present in children with cerebral palsy long after the normal time when these reflexes should have disappeared. The persistence of the tonic neck reflex will interfere with normal motor function. Each time the child turns his head his body will involuntarily move into the obligatory posture of the tonic neck reflex and thus prevent normal coordinated motor functions. These problems must be overcome if the child is to develop motor skills.

Any discussion of cerebral palsy must begin with definitions of the multitude of terms used to describe motor abnormalities. With regard to muscle weakness, the term "plegia" refers to complete paralysis of muscles whereas "paresis" refers to partial paralysis; that is, weakness but not total inability to use the muscles. Spasticity is an increase in tone of a muscle due to upper motor neuron damage (see Chap. 13), resulting in release of inhibitory influences on the muscle. Muscles are affected to different degrees in spastic weakness. In the arms, muscles of flexion are stronger than muscles of extension, so the characteristic posture of an arm with spastic paralysis is flexion of all the joints with a closed or fisted hand. In the legs, the muscles of extension are stronger than the muscles of flexion, and the typical posture of spastic weakness in the lower extremity is extension of all joints.

Hypotonia is decrease in muscle tone, resulting in "floppiness" or flaccid muscles. When used in relation to cerebral palsy, hypotonia usually is related to cerebellar damage.

The patterns of weakness seen in cerebral palsy are described in Table 9–1.

Other forms of cerebral palsy include choreoathetoid, ataxic and mixed types. Choreoathetoid cerebral palsy presents primarily as a movement disorder with uncontrollable jerking and writhing movements of the extremities and sometimes of

TABLE 9–1.—PATTERNS OF WEAKNESS IN CEREBRAL PALSY

Monoplegia—paralysis of one limb only
Hemiplegia—paralysis of arm and leg on same side of body
Diplegia—paralysis of both legs *or* both arms
Paraplegia—paralysis of both legs
Quadriplegia—paralysis of all four limbs

the trunk. Other forms of involuntary movements (for example, dystonia) often are seen as well (see Chap. 2 for description of involuntary movements). Ataxia refers to lack of coordination because of cerebellar damage. Truncal ataxia produces inability to maintain balance and causes a "drunken" gait, with staggering or falling to one side. Ataxia of the limbs causes inability to reach directly for an object without knocking it over. In mixed types of cerebral palsy, two or more of the above abnormalities are seen in the same patient.

DIAGNOSIS OF CEREBRAL PALSY

Children with severe neurologic handicaps secondary to perinatal difficulties present no problem in diagnosis. They usually have severely delayed motor milestones and show evidence of spasticity and lack of muscle coordination. In addition, they may have seizures and mental retardation. The diagnosis can be made by obtaining a history of some difficulty in the perinatal period and of delayed developmental milestones with no indication of regression of milestones. Diagnosis may be more difficult in mild cases of motor dysfunction. Often an infant with cerebral palsy first comes to the attention of a physician because the parents have noticed a delay in development of motor milestones. Depending on the type of cerebral palsy, only some motor functions may be impaired; for example, the child may use his hands appropriately but not his legs. In extremely mild cases there may be no detectable problem except that, for example, the child's walking might be delayed a few months. When the child does start to walk, the parents may notice that he walks on his toes.

Intellectual impairment is not a necessary component of cerebral palsy, but in cases of generalized and severe brain damage, mental retardation may be present as well as motor problems. Likewise, seizures may occur as a component of cerebral palsy but are not an invariable feature.

There is no laboratory test that can diagnose or exclude the presence of cerebral palsy. Diagnosis is based on the neurologic examination, and, if necessary, exclusion of progressive diseases should be done by appropriate laboratory tests (see Chap. 8).

SPASTIC QUADRIPLEGIA

This type of motor deficit was the original problem described by Little in 1861 (cerebral palsy has also been referred to as Little's disease). Spastic quadriplegia describes impairment of function in all four extremities, with weakness and tightness or rigidity of muscles due to increased tone. The legs typically are more impaired than the arms; coordinated functions such as walking and reaching for objects may be ex-

Fig. 9–1.—A 10-month-old infant with spastic quadriplegia, demonstrating typical posture of flexion in the upper extremities with the hands held in fisted positions. Usual lower-extremity posture of hyperextension is not prominent in this patient.

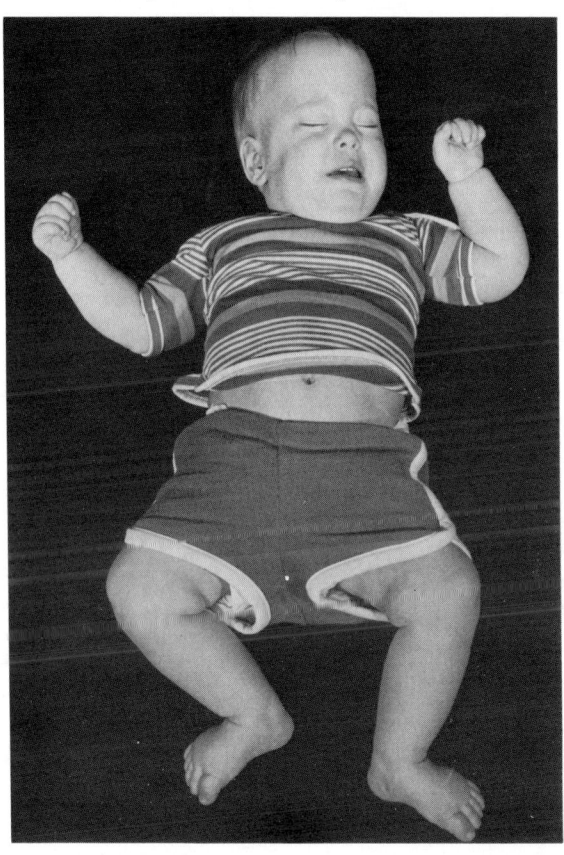

tremely difficult to achieve because of this spasticity. Clearly articulated speech and coordinated swallowing may also be impaired because of bilateral cerebral damage, which produces a "pseudobulbar palsy." Drooling often is a significant problem in these children.

The typical posture of infants with spastic quadriplegia is flexion of the upper extremities with the hands held tightly fisted whereas the legs are hyperextended and difficult to flex (Fig. 9–1).

Mental retardation is relatively common with this type of cerebral palsy and seizures occur in approximately 50% of such patients.

Significant spasticity often is accompanied by clonus, which is a rapid, rhythmic, jerking or flexion/extension of a part of the body, most commonly the ankle. Clonus can be elicited by briskly flexing the ankle; this initiates repetitive beats of clonus that can be felt and seen by the examiner. In severe cases, clonus may appear spontaneously, especially when slight pressure is applied to the foot, as when the child attempts to stand. Clonus can be so frequently and easily produced that it makes attempts at walking impossible.

SPASTIC DIPLEGIA

This type of cerebral palsy is found most often in infants who were premature; the reason for this is not clear. Spastic diplegia refers to weakness and increase in tone in both arms *or* both legs; in most cases, the legs are involved. These children may have normal developmental milestones in the first few months—for example, rolling over, reaching for objects and sitting—but walking may be delayed. On examination there is increased tone in the lower extremities and increased deep tendon reflexes, the thighs may be held adducted (pulled toward each other) and the legs are extended. When the child is suspended upright by supporting him under the arms, the legs tend to cross because of tightness in the adductors. This posture is called scissoring.

When children with spastic diplegia do begin to walk, they may walk on their toes. Gait often is clumsy and lacks normal

coordination. Under stress, such
tures such as arm flexion or lack
come apparent. Children with s
significant intellectual impair
also normal.

Atonic diplegia is a variar
fants with cerebral palsy, i
legs yet deep tendon refle?
these infants get older, tone
affected limbs. The reason for the dec.
of problem is not clear.

SPASTIC HEMIPLEGIA

Weakness of one side of the body probably is a result of at least two separate causes. The first is a stroke, or infarct, that occurs during intrauterine development because of maldevelopment of one of the blood vessels inside the head. A second cause is a vascular accident or stroke that occurs in early infancy (acute infantile hemiplegia). There are several underlying mechanisms that may produce acute infantile hemiplegia, including infections, severe seizures and significant head trauma.

Whatever the event that produced the hemiplegia, the patients exhibit similar problems. These include weakness of the arm and the leg on the same side of the body and increased tone in the limbs. The characteristic posture of these children is flexion of the arm, with the hand held in a closed or fisted position, and extension of the leg (Fig. 9-2). These children may have delayed motor milestones because they lack the symmetric strength needed for truncal stability. Thus, for example, when the child is placed in a seated position, he tends to fall to the weak side. When walking begins, the child may drag the weak leg or walk on his toes on the affected side. The characteristic gait of a hemiplegic child is that of circumduction of the weak leg; that is, the weak leg is thrown out and brought slowly back in.

Children with hemiplegia tend to show hand preference very early, using the strong hand for most tasks, as opposed to

CEREBRAL PALSY

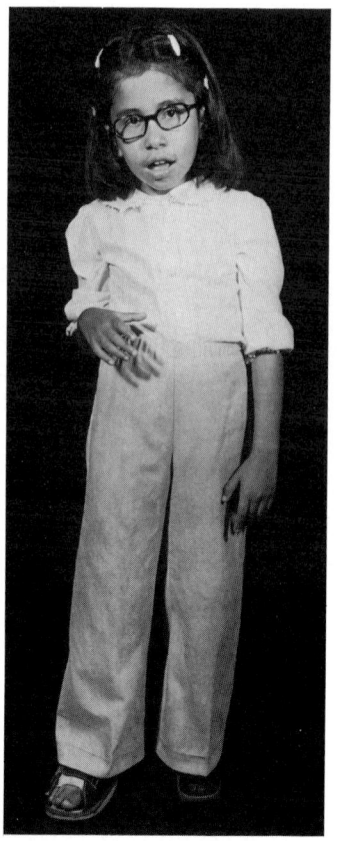

Fig. 9–2.—A child with spastic hemiplegia secondary to brain tumor. Note posture of flexion in the right arm and brace on right foot.

a normal infant, who utilizes both hands for tasks and does not show strong dominance before 2 or 3 years of age. Arm swing during walking is absent on the weak side and often the weak arm is held flexed. Absence of normal cerebral control of arm and leg function also results in lack of appropriate growth of these limbs, so that in hemiplegic children, the affected leg and arm often will be smaller than the normal side (Fig. 9–3). A high percentage of these children also have seizure disorders, often focal motor in type, with seizure activity (tonic and/or clonic movements) involving only the weak side.

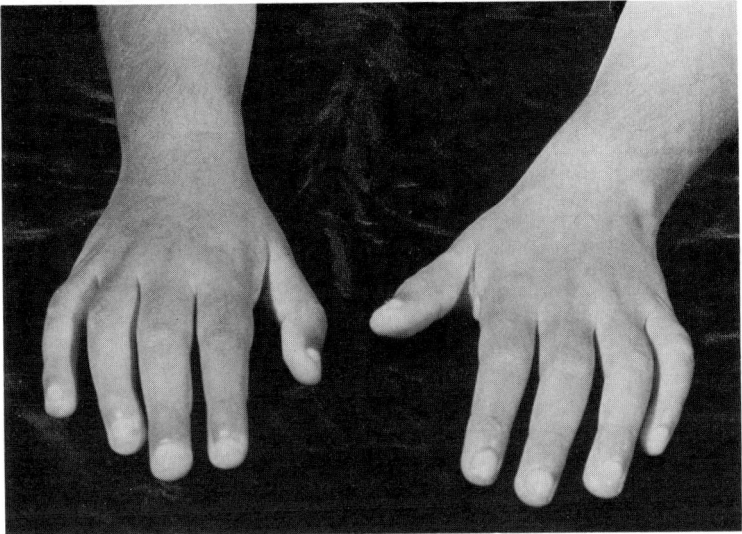

Fig. 9-3.—Comparison of size of hands in a patient with spastic hemiplegia. The right hand is noticeably smaller than the left.

CHOREOATHETOID CEREBRAL PALSY

Damage to certain parts of the brain (especially the basal ganglia) results in lack of coordinated voluntary movements and in abnormal movements. Some infants who have sustained brain damage secondary to lack of oxygen (anoxia) develop this type of cerebral palsy. Choreoathetosis is a combination of two abnormal types of movements—chorea, or quick jerky movements of large parts of the extremities, and athetosis, or slow writhing movements of more distal parts of the body. These children have great difficulty in coordinating body movements to walk, reach for objects, etc. They also have difficulty with clear articulation of speech and with swallowing because of abnormalities of oral musculature.

Children with choreoathetoid cerebral palsy often have spasticity as well, which further impairs functional ability. When severe anoxia is the cause of these problems, intellectual function may be impaired as well.

One specific cause of choreoathetosis is kernicterus. This disorder is the result of severe jaundice in the neonatal period; for example, from Rh blood group incompatibility between mother and child. Jaundice, or yellow discoloration of the skin, is caused by an excess of a pigment called bilirubin. One form of bilirubin readily crosses from blood into brain and is deposited preferentially in certain parts of the brain, producing damage to those areas.

Infants with kernicterus initially are lethargic, with decreased tone and poor suck. Over the first 2 years of life they exhibit choreoathetosis and increased muscle tone. Hearing impairment is common as well.

Kernicterus can be prevented in many instances by careful attention to the concentration of bilirubin in the blood. In general, bilirubin should not rise above 15 mg/100 ml in premature infants and 20 mg/100 ml in full-term infants. If bilirubin levels approach these numbers, infants should be placed under a special light. In severe cases, exchange blood transfusions may be necessary to decrease bilirubin concentrations.

APPROACH TO THERAPY OF PATIENTS WITH CEREBRAL PALSY

Classifications for cerebral palsy based on the degree of functional impairment have been suggested: the mildest group, or Class I — minimal limitation of activity; Class II — mild to moderate limitation; Class III — moderate to severe limitation; and Class IV — inability to perform any useful motor functions. This system has its primary usefulness in terms of longitudinal evaluations of the patient before and during therapy.

Other than anticonvulsant medication in patients with seizure disorders, few drugs are beneficial in treating the manifestations of cerebral palsy. Two medications have been useful in decreasing spasticity when this complication is so severe as to be detrimental to useful function or to rehabilitative efforts. Diazepam (Valium) is quite effective in reducing spasticity and has been of value to many patients. The primary side effect of diazepam is drowsiness, and the dose may need to be reduced if drowsiness is significant. A newer drug called dantrolene (Dantrium) has also proved to be effective in reducing spasticity in many patients, but its use in children is not widespread as yet. Major side effects of dantrolene include drowsiness and the potential for liver damage. Therefore, this drug must be used with caution.

REHABILITATIVE THERAPY

A combined approach by physical, occupational and speech therapists should be initiated early in children with manifestations of cerebral palsy. This is true even in patients with mild forms, so that they do not develop compensatory habits. In early infancy, range of motion exercises may be the primary form of treatment. Physical and occupational therapy programs should be directed toward inhibition of abnormal muscle tone and primitive reflexes and facilitation of normal motor patterns. As early as possible, these children should begin programs to improve balance, truncal stability and head control, working on developmental progression to sitting, standing, walking and oral stimulation exercises through inhibition and facilitation. Parents should be taught how to handle the child and should be encouraged to take an active part in the total treatment program. Children with severe handicaps may need many years of combined therapy before any useful function is achieved.

ORTHOPEDIC DEVICES

It is important for all infants to have appropriate visual, auditory and tactile stimuli to increase alertness and interest in the environment. This is even more imperative for children with handicaps. Yet, infants with poor motor function too often are left to lie in a crib most of the day because they lack the control to sit in an infant seat. A specially designed infant seat with padding on the sides to prevent falling out and with head guards to keep the head from falling to one side can be devised to fit the individual child and allow him to "sit up" much of the time. The chair should be tilted back about 30 degrees

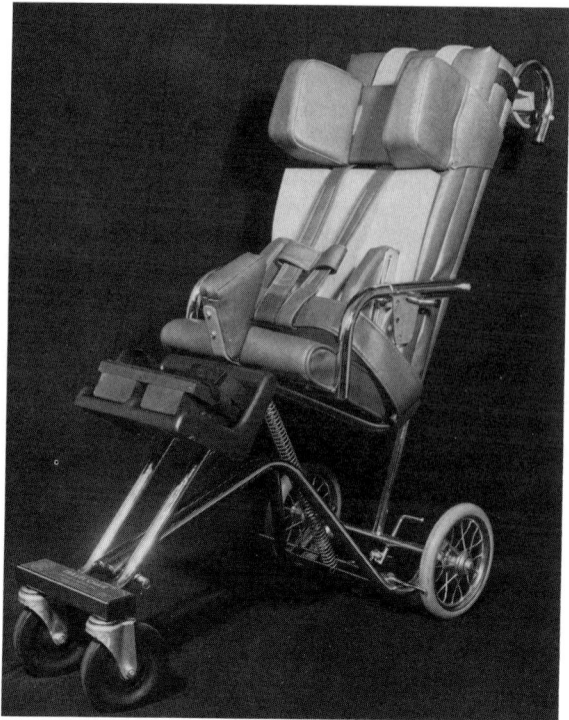

Fig. 9–4.—Specially designed chair for infant with multiple motor problems. Chair is tilted back to help support head; headrests prevent head from falling to the side; harness holds child in place; scoliosis pads (on lower chair back) prevent poor posture. Back wheels can be lifted up so that chair fits on car seat. Tray can be attached to arms of chair.

so that the head can rest on the back and does not fall forward. For older children with severe motor handicaps, a similarly designed wheelchair can be useful (Figs. 9–4 and 9–5).

Children with spastic hemiplegia often have one leg shorter than the other. This asymmetry produces a limp, which aggravates the gait abnormality further. An orthopedic shoe with a raised sole will equalize the length of the two legs and permit improvement in walking. Braces may also be helpful in improving joint stability in a weak leg.

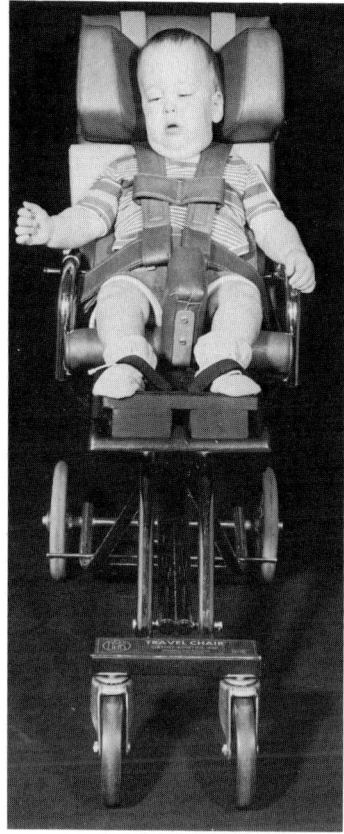

Fig. 9–5. — Infant with spastic quadriplegia in chair fitted for him.

SURGERY

Over a period of time, severe spasticity can result in fixed positions of the limbs, which produces severe limitation of movement. In some cases, surgical intervention to cut the tendon of an involved muscle can decrease spasticity and improve mobility. For example, prolonged extension of the foot may produce a contracture at the ankle (heel cord tightening), which makes it impossible to flex the ankle. Surgically cutting the Achilles tendon will reduce the spasticity and allow flexion of the foot to be restored.

PROGNOSIS

Many children with cerebral palsy are minimally impaired and can lead a totally normal life. Even children with moderate to severe neurologic impairment initially can improve to the stage of very adequate function. Early initiation of a multifaceted rehabilitative and educational program can improve such a child's functional ability greatly. Parents should have thorough counseling about their child's problem. They should be informed that cerebral palsy does *not* get worse, that in many instances the child's neurologic function will improve, and that intellectual function may be normal. With this information parents tend to have a more optimistic outlook and to cooperate well with rehabilitation efforts.

10

NERVE AND MUSCLE DISEASES

IN ORDER FOR normal strength and muscle coordination to occur, all components of the neuromuscular system must be functional. The *motor unit* is the integrated circuit that is responsible for muscle activity. Each motor unit consists of a nerve cell or anterior horn cell in the spinal cord, the nerve fiber projections of that cell, the neuromuscular junction connecting the fiber to the muscle and all of the muscle fibers that that nerve cell innervates (Fig. 10-1). Damage to any part of the motor unit can produce weakness or decrease in functional ability of the muscle. Muscle weakness may occur in all or most muscles (generalized weakness) or may be present in only a few muscles. Distribution of weakness may be random (patchy weakness) or may have a specific pattern. Proximal

Fig. 10–1.—Schematic representation of a motor unit.

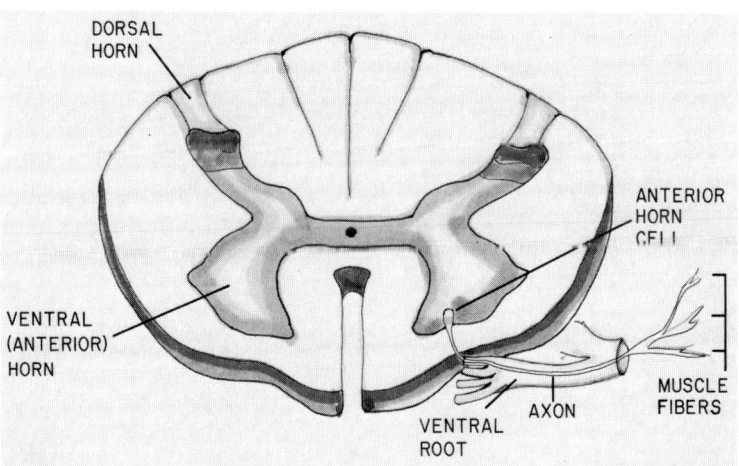

weakness affects muscles of the trunk or close to the trunk (e.g., shoulders, thighs) whereas distal weakness occurs in muscles farthest from the trunk (feet, hands). If a nerve is damaged, the injury is called a *neuropathy*. A *myopathy* exists if the muscle itself is damaged. Certain diseases can damage the connection between nerve and muscle, called the *neuromuscular junction*. This chapter will deal with diseases that affect various segments of the motor unit.

ANTERIOR HORN CELL DISEASES

Nerve cells that innervate muscles are located in the ventral horn of the spinal cord and are called *anterior horn cells* or *lower motor neurons*. Anterior horn cells, in turn, receive impulses from nerve cells in the motor areas of the brain *(upper motor neurons)* as well as from other areas. If damage to a lower motor neuron occurs, the result is muscle weakness, decreased tone in the muscle, absence of normal reflexes and muscle atrophy. For unclear reasons, certain diseases have a predilection for anterior horn cells and can produce selective damage to these cells. *Poliomyelitis* (infantile paralysis) is a classic example of a disease that selectively destroys anterior horn cells. This disease is caused by a virus that gets into the spinal cord and attacks anterior horn cells. Damage may not be uniform throughout the spinal cord, however, so that weakness may develop in only one part of the body if the virus primarily attacks cells in that area. Thus, for example, some people afflicted with polio may develop weakness of a leg only. When damage is widespread, on the other hand, diffuse weakness can result, including paralysis of muscles required for breathing. In the past, before polio was controlled by immunization, children with widespread polio often required special mechanical respirators ("iron lungs") to breathe, since their own respiratory muscles were too weak.

Once a polio infection is contracted there is no cure. Treatment consists primarily of physical therapy aimed at preventing contractures and gait retraining if only partial weakness occurs. Fortunately, with the advent of the Salk and then Sabin antipolio vaccines, this disease now is extremely uncom-

Anterior Horn Cell Diseases

mon in the United States. However, the virus has not eradicated and failure to vaccinate children could result resurgence of paralytic polio cases.

Other viral infections can mimic polio but few have such devastating results.

A group of hereditary disorders, called the *spinal muscular atrophies*, also specifically affect anterior horn cells and produce generalized weakness. An infantile form, called Werdnig-Hoffmann disease, has its onset at birth with generalized weakness, poor muscle tone, weak cry and poor suck. This disease is inherited as an autosomal recessive disorder. It is progressive, with steadily increasing weakness, and affected infants usually die in the first year or two of life from respiratory failure. Unfortunately, there is no effective treatment as yet for this disease.

A milder form of hereditary spinal muscular atrophy, Kugelberg-Welander syndrome, has its onset in later childhood, with slow development of muscle weakness. These children generally are not as severely affected as those with the infantile form and can lead relatively normal lives for many years. The majority of children with this disease, however, will be unable to walk by the late teens or early twenties.

There is no cure for these disorders. However, a good physical therapy program can help greatly to prevent contractures and to strengthen unaffected muscles so that the child will be able to remain ambulatory for a longer period. Since the anterior horn cells are damaged in a patchy fashion, a thorough physical therapy evaluation can determine which muscles still are strong and therapy can be designed to strengthen those muscles and to train the patient to rely on those muscles for walking and other self-care functions.

Amyotrophic lateral sclerosis (ALS, Lou Gehrig's disease) is a crippling and usually fatal disease of unknown cause that produces destruction of the motor neurons almost exclusively. ALS usually is not hereditary. Most patients with ALS develop the disease as adults, but there are a few cases in which the illness develops in the teenage years. Progressive muscle weakness and atrophy develop, and patients may require respiratory assistance. At present, there is no effective treatment for ALS, and therapy is primarily supportive, aimed at preventing contractures and mobilizing the patient as much as possible.

DISORDERS OF PERIPHERAL NERVES

The peripheral nerves are made up of long projections from the nerve cell bodies that connect the cells in the spinal cord with the muscles. Most of these nerve fibers *(axons)* are covered with a sheath called *myelin*. Myelin aids in the rapid transmission of electrical impulses from the cell body to the neuromuscular junction. These impulses are the means by which the nerve cells send messages to other parts of the body. When the electrical impulse reaches the neuromuscular junction, it "instructs" the nerve terminal to release small amounts of a chemical (acetylcholine), which goes to the muscle side of the junction and causes the muscle to begin a process of contraction. In this way, the nerve controls muscle function.

If the axon or the myelin sheath is damaged, the ability to transmit electrical impulses is impaired and weakness can result, not because of muscle damage but because the muscle does not receive the proper instructions from the nerve. When such damage occurs, it is called *peripheral neuropathy*. Peripheral neuropathies tend to affect distal body parts first, so that hands and feet would be expected to be more involved than shoulders and thighs.

Many agents are toxic to the nerve fiber or to myelin. Chronic lead and arsenic poisoning as well as other environmental toxins can lead to a peripheral neuropathy. Symptoms may include weakness, decreased or absent reflexes such as the knee jerk and sensory abnormalities such as tingling, burning or numbness in the hands or feet. The damage caused by toxic agents is insidious and becomes obvious only after prolonged or repeated exposure to the toxin. Continued heavy exposure to alcohol in adolescents and adults can also produce a painful peripheral neuropathy. Diphenylhydantoin, a frequently prescribed anticonvulsant, when taken over a period of many years, can also cause peripheral nerve damage. In this case,

Disorders of Peripheral Nerves

however, the neuropathy is very mild and usually is found only on careful neurologic examination.

Certain infectious agents can cause a peripheral neuropathy as well as producing symptoms elsewhere in the body. Among the viral diseases involving peripheral nerves are infectious hepatitis, mumps and mononucleosis. Bacterial infections such as diphtheria and leprosy may also produce peripheral neuropathies. With these infectious diseases, other symptoms usually are present as well. The exception is leprosy, which is rare in most of the United States but still occurs in certain parts of the country. The organism responsible for leprosy can produce a peripheral neuropathy without much symptomatology elsewhere in the body. Treatment of the peripheral nerve disturbance is based on treatment of the underlying infection where possible.

One form of inflammation of peripheral nerves occurring after infections is called *Guillain-Barré syndrome*, or postinfectious polyneuritis. Guillain-Barré syndrome follows certain viral infections and recently has been reported following administration of influenza vaccine. Inflammation of the myelin sheaths is the pathologic abnormality. The illness is characterized by an ascending paralysis; i.e., weakness usually begins in the feet and moves slowly upward over the course of days to weeks. The paralysis may stop anywhere in the body; if total, it can involve the muscles of respiration and require mechanical support (respirators) to maintain breathing. Once the inflammatory response has subsided, strength usually returns, with the first involved muscles being the last to regain strength.

Guillain-Barré syndrome can occur in any age group, and without appropriate respiratory support can be fatal. However, with close medical supervision, the prognosis is quite good in most cases. Treatment consists primarily of respiratory support, good chest physiotherapy to prevent pneumonia and physical therapy to prevent contractures in paralyzed muscles. Administration of steroid hormones may shorten the course of the illness. As the patient recovers strength, a comprehensive program of physical and occupational therapy should be instituted to aid in return of useful muscle function.

Long-term deficiency of certain vitamins, especially B_1, B_6 and B_{12}, can lead to peripheral neuropathies. These deficiencies can be due to inadequate dietary intake or to inability of the gastrointestinal tract to absorb a particular vitamin. Treatment is based on replacement of the appropriate vitamin.

Peripheral neuropathies may be an accompanying symptom of some metabolic diseases and may, in fact, form the patient's only complaint. Hypothyroidism, chronic liver and kidney failure and diabetes mellitus can have peripheral neuropathy as a prominent symptom. In the case of diabetes and the collagen vascular diseases (systemic lupus erythematosus, polyarteritis nodosa), blood vessels supplying nutrients to the nerves become blocked and nerve damage occurs as a result of lack of blood supply. In these cases, onset of symptoms may be very sudden, unlike most causes of peripheral neuropathy, which require many weeks or months to appear.

Treatment is based on the underlying disease. Symptoms of diabetic peripheral neuropathy can be minimized by good control of blood sugar. Hypothyroidism requires thyroid hormone replacement therapy. Collagen vascular diseases often respond to steroid hormone treatment.

Finally, some rare hereditary diseases can affect peripheral nerves but are accompanied by signs of other nervous system dysfunction as well. There usually is a family history of similar symptoms. Specific treatment is available for a few of these.

DISEASES OF THE NEUROMUSCULAR JUNCTION

The *neuromuscular junction* is the gap between nerve and muscle. Electrical impulses from the nerve travel to the neuromuscular junction and cause release (from the presynaptic membrane) of the chemical neurotransmitter *acetylcholine*. Acetylcholine then alters the muscle (postsynaptic) membrane in such a way as to cause an electrical impulse, which, in turn, produces a coordinated contraction of the muscle fiber. Diseases that damage the neuromuscular junction do so in one of several ways. They may decrease the number of packets of acetylcholine released on the presynaptic side or interfere with the reception of acetylcholine on the postsynaptic membrane.

Botulism is an infectious disease caused by bacteria that grow in inadequately prepared canned foods. Once inside the body, these bacteria release a toxin that selectively attacks the neuromuscular junction on the presynaptic side and prevents release of acetylcholine. Symptoms begin within 18–36 hours after eating contaminated food. Progressive and generalized weakness (including facial and oral weakness) occurs and can lead to respiratory paralysis. Death can ensue if respiratory function is not supported by mechanical respirators. Treatment consists primarily of thorough respiratory care. After the illness has reached its maximal severity, recovery proceeds gradually, with strength increasing over a period of weeks to months. As strength improves, comprehensive physical, occupational and speech therapy programs are useful adjuncts to help maximal return of function.

Recently, several cases of infantile botulism have been reported in certain areas of the United States. This problem had not been recognized previously as a cause of symptoms in infants. The syndrome of infantile botulism consists of a subtle progression of muscle weakness accompanied by constipation in a previously well infant. These children tend to lose the ability to hold the head upright as one of the first symptoms of muscle weakness. The illness can progress to respiratory difficulties and, at times, the children will need ventilatory support. These infants require hospitalization and intensive supportive care during the acute illness, but strength gradually returns over a period of days to weeks. Infantile botulism can mimic the symptoms of Guillain-Barré syndrome, but the spores of the botulism organism can be isolated from the stool of infants infected with this disease. The outlook for recovery in these children is quite good with the proper supportive therapy.

Myasthenia gravis is a disorder that also involves the neuromuscular junction. It is characterized by weakness of voluntary muscles anywhere in the body, especially after activity, with strength returning after a rest period. Weakness may vary greatly in different muscles. The cause of myasthenia gravis is not known but is thought to involve an attack on the junction by the body's immune system. Circulating antibodies to the postsynaptic receptor can be detected in the blood of many patients with myasthenia gravis. The site of the abnormality is the postsynaptic side of the neuromuscular junction, where a membrane receptor that normally reacts with acetylcholine appears to be missing or malfunctioning. The characteristic clinical symptom is excessive fatigability of muscles after exercise. Treatment is based on pharmacologically increasing the amount of acetylcholine available to the receptors. This may be accomplished by administration of drugs known as cholinesterase inhibitors (edrophonium, neostigmine, physostigmine). Another approach to therapy involves attempts to suppress formation of antibodies to muscle receptors by administration of the corticosteroid prednisone. A surgical procedure to remove the thymus gland has also led to improvement in some cases of myasthenia gravis.

There appear to be three separate clinical presentations of myasthenia gravis in childhood. *Transient neonatal myasthenia* may occur in infants born to mothers with myasthenia gravis. Such infants become weak soon after birth, at times within a few hours, and the symptoms follow a pattern of rapidly worsening weakness over several days to weeks, followed by gradual improvement. These infants may be so weak that they cannot suck adequately; crying may be poor and respiratory distress is a possible problem. Adequate respiratory and supportive care (for example, chest physical therapy and intravenous or nasogastric tube feedings) are essential for survival during this period. Children with transient neonatal myasthenia usually recover completely by 4–6 weeks of age and require no further treatment. There is no firm evidence to suggest that these children will develop the more chronic form of the disease later.

The second presentation of this problem in children is *congenital myasthenia*. Unlike transient neonatal myasthenia, infants with congenital myasthenia are not born to mothers with the disease; however, there appears to be a familial tendency to myasthenia gravis in such cases. These infants have symptoms beginning soon after birth. Weakness predominates in the muscles of eye movement and facial movement, with less involvement of other parts of the body. Diagnosis is made by giving an injection of a small amount of the anticholinesterase edrophonium and observing rapid improvement in strength. Electrical recordings from muscles (electromyography) can also be used to help confirm the diagnosis.

Treatment consists of daily oral administration of one of the anticholinesterase drugs. These drugs have a short duration of action and usually must be taken every 4 hours. As the drug effect wears off, most patients with myasthenia become noticeably weaker.

A third form of this disease is *juvenile myasthenia.* This form of myasthenia gravis is similar to that seen in adults. Onset usually is after 1 year of age and may be associated with weakness anywhere in the body. However, most children with juvenile myasthenia will have drooping of the eyelids (ptosis) or double vision (diplopia) as early symptoms. Some children will go on to develop weakness of respiratory muscles, which can be life-threatening. Others (approximately 20%) will have a spontaneous remission of all symptoms for an indefinite period.

Diagnosis is confirmed as for congenital myasthenia by injecting edrophonium intravenously and observing improvement in strength. Electromyographic abnormalities are confirmatory also.

Treatment usually is begun with one of the anticholinesterase agents or with prednisone if the former drug fails to achieve adequate improvement. Early thymectomy is advocated for children with severe or generalized myasthenia gravis or in whom drug therapy fails.

The prognosis for patients with myasthenia gravis depends on the type of muscles involved, the severity of the disease and the response to the above modes of therapy. Some children achieve a permanent remission of symptoms; in others, the disease may stabilize at some level of disability; still others have a chronically progressive course with serious complications.

When muscles of the face and mouth are severely involved

(bulbar palsy), patients may have significant problems with chewing, swallowing, speaking and handling saliva effectively. Speech is impaired and drooling may occur. Speech and occupational therapy can be useful when the problem is not too severe. Such therapy certainly should be tried in these patients.

The Myasthenia Gravis Foundation is a national organization that seeks to inform patients about their illness through informative brochures and to raise funds for research. Parents of such patients can contact the foundation through its national headquarters located at 230 Park Avenue, New York, New York, 10017.

MUSCLE DISEASES

Disorders that produce damage to the muscles directly are called myopathies. The muscular dystrophies are a group of primary muscle diseases that are *inherited* and in which the muscle weakness becomes progressively more severe with age. Some children are born with muscle weakness caused by some developmental or chemical abnormalities in the muscle; these children are said to have congenital myopathies.

MUSCULAR DYSTROPHY. — There are several types of muscular dystrophy, differentiated by type of inheritance, age at onset of first symptoms and rapidity of disease progression. The most common types are outlined in Table 10–1. In the more severe forms of muscular dystrophy, such as Duchenne's,

TABLE 10–1. — THE MUSCULAR DYSTROPHIES

TYPE	MODE OF INHERITANCE	USUAL AGE AT ONSET OF SYMPTOMS	RATE OF PROGRESSION
Duchenne	X-linked recessive	2–4 years	Rapid
Becker	X-linked recessive	After 6 years	Slow to moderate
Myotonic	Autosomal dominant	Variable	Variable
Facioscapulohumeral	Autosomal dominant	7–25 years	Slow
Limb-girdle	Autosomal recessive and sporadic	Variable	Variable

weakness becomes noticeable by the age of 3 years in most cases, and these children develop progressive muscle wasting, weakness, contractures and spinal deformities. They usually are confined to a wheelchair by the time of adolescence. Life expectancy is shortened because of progressive weakness of muscles used for moving the chest wall and breathing and because of involvement of the heart muscle.

Diagnosis is made by a combination of several tests and clinical criteria. Blood concentrations of muscle enzymes (creatine phosphokinase, aldolase) can be measured and are elevated in Duchenne's dystrophy. Clinically, muscles of the calf initially appear larger than normal for age, a condition referred to as "pseudohypertrophy." Surgical biopsy for microscopic examination of a weak muscle reveals reduction in the number of muscle fibers, degeneration of fibers, great irregularity in the size of muscle fibers, with some abnormally small ones scattered among unusually enlarged ones, and an increase in fat and connective tissue surrounding the muscle fibers.

Each type of muscular dystrophy has typical clinical patterns of weakness that are useful diagnostically. These patterns are combined with a family history and the laboratory tests mentioned above to make the diagnosis.

There is no curative treatment as yet for muscular dystrophy. Therapy is directed at prevention of contractures by physical therapy, correction of spinal deformities when possible (e.g., with braces) and the use of crutches or walkers to maintain mobility for as long as possible. Although the long-term outlook for children with severe forms of muscular dystrophy is poor, those with milder forms may lead active lives for many years. All deserve the benefit of a well-planned physical therapy program to maximize mobility and independence.

The Muscular Dystrophy Association, a nationwide organization, seeks to provide children affected with muscular dystrophy and other muscle diseases with a comprehensive program of medical and rehabilitative therapy. Summer camp programs are available for these children in many areas of the country, and parents should be advised to contact the Muscular Dystrophy Association's national office at 810 Seventh Avenue, New York, New York 10019 for details regarding facilities in their area.

CONGENITAL MYOPATHIES.—These are a group of diseases that usually cause muscle weakness and hypotonia ("floppiness") in infancy. Some cases appear to be familial but many are not. These disorders are classified primarily on the basis of the abnormality seen on microscopic examination of the muscle. Clinical features are diverse, ranging from eventually normal strength to severe weakness. Diagnosis is based on microscopic examination of a weak muscle. In general there is no effective treatment for this group of diseases. However, the outlook is good for spontaneous improvement or at least lack of progressive weakness in many instances.

ACQUIRED MYOPATHIES.—Muscle weakness may be the only or primary symptom in a variety of diseases, and certain drugs and chemicals can produce myopathic symptoms.

Hyperthyroidism can cause weakness, particularly in proximal parts of arms and legs, sometimes with diminution in size of the affected muscles. Unlike the congenital or primary myopathies, microscopic examination of a weak muscle secondary to hyperthyroidism often is normal. In a previously healthy person with recent onset of muscle weakness, thyroid disease should be suspected. Diagnosis can be made by obtaining blood for a thyroxine level. Treatment of the hyperthyroid problem can alleviate the symptoms of the myopathy.

Hypothyroidism in children can also cause muscle abnormalities, including weakness, painful muscle cramps and unusual enlargement of muscle groups. Treatment of the underlying disease with thyroid hormone replacement produces alleviation of the muscle symptoms.

A group of disorders called collagen vascular diseases, including systemic lupus erythematosus, may produce symptoms in multiple organs, including kidney, skin and nervous system. They may also cause a myopathy (at times painful) of proximal muscles. These symptoms often disappear with steroid hormone treatment; such treatment may also alleviate symptoms in other involved organs.

One specific form of collagen disease, polymyositis, affects muscles preferentially. This disorder can occur at any age, although it is uncommon in children. Symptoms include progressive proximal muscle weakness, and at times the muscles are unusually firm and painful to touch. The weakness may also affect the muscles of the face and the oral musculature, and children with this disorder may have difficulty swallowing.

Diagnosis is at times difficult to establish, and is made by finding an elevated erythrocyte sedimentation rate, elevations of CPK, and by muscle biopsy which shows an inflammatory reaction around blood vessels inside the muscles.

Treatment consists of the oral administration of steroid hormones. The prognosis is variable in children, but sometimes the disease goes into remission during steroid therapy and the patient may be symptom free for many years.

The outlook for the acquired myopathies depends in part on the severity of the underlying disease. In many cases, effective treatment of the primary disorder will produce alleviation of the myopathic symptoms as well.

II

INFECTIONS OF THE CENTRAL NERVOUS SYSTEM

INFECTIOUS AGENTS can invade the central nervous system and produce infection in the brain and its surrounding membranes. Routes of entry of infection into the brain include the blood (carrying infection from elsewhere in the body), sinuses, nose, ears and skin. Children who have fractures of the skull can develop central nervous system infections from direct spread of a microorganism from the surface; for example, through the nose, since there is no barrier protecting the nervous system at the fracture point.

The nervous system responds to infection in a limited variety of ways. Inflammation of the protective membranes of the brain is called *meningitis*. Diffuse infection of the brain itself also results in an inflammatory response referred to as *encephalitis*. A combination of the two sites of inflammation is known as *meningoencephalitis*. An area of inflammation also may be localized to a single segment of brain, and purulent material, or pus, can form within this area; this is called a *brain abscess*. Meningitis, encephalitis and brain abscess are the three major categories of central nervous system infections.

Various pathogenic and relatively nonpathogenic microorganisms can infect the nervous system, but the common agents are bacteria, viruses and fungi. Diagnosis, treatment and outcome depend on the type of microorganism, its virulence and its responsiveness to treatment.

MENINGITIS

Symptoms and signs of meningitis depend on the age of the patient. In an infant under a year of age, symptoms usually are

MENINGITIS

nonspecific: fever, poor feeding, irritability, lethargy, vomiting or seizures may be the only clinical signs. On examination, the *fontanelle* (soft spot on the top of the head) may be bulging or tense. In older children, more specific clinical signs can be detected. The most characteristic sign is a *stiff neck* due to irritation of the meninges. Pain induced by movement of the head or neck causes the child to guard these parts of the body and hold them relatively immobile. Other symptoms in the older child include sensitivity of the eyes to light *(photophobia)*, headache, irritability and lethargy. Seizures may occur in all age groups. Increased pressure inside the head causes swelling of the optic nerve in back of the eye; this can be detected, when present, during the course of a careful examination of the patient's eyes by the physician.

The only definitive way to diagnose meningitis is through analysis of the cerebrospinal fluid obtained by performing a lumbar puncture or spinal tap. This procedure is accomplished by inserting a special needle through the skin of the lower back and into the sac of fluid that surrounds the spinal cord and nerve roots. One to two teaspoonfuls (5–10 ml) of spinal fluid are removed through the needle and the needle is then withdrawn. The fluid is examined under the microscope for the presence of cells and bacteria and analyzed biochemically for concentrations of protein and glucose. In the presence of meningitis there is an increased number of cells in the spinal fluid as well as an increase in the protein content and a decrease in the glucose concentration when compared to the amount of glucose in the blood. Using this type of analysis, the diagnosis of meningitis can readily be made.

Meningitis usually is one of three major types, classified on the basis of the causative microorganism: bacterial, viral or fungal. Other infectious agents, including rickettsiae and protozoa, are also infrequent causes of meningitis.

BACTERIAL INFECTIONS.—Certain bacteria are more commonly found in specific age groups (Table 11–1). Since each organism responds to a specific antibiotic, it is important to identify the infectious agent early for effective treatment. Several types of bacteria have a predilection for newborn infants. These include streptococcus group B, *Staphylococcus aureus*

TABLE 11-1.—PRIMARY TYPES OF BACTERIAL MENINGITIS IN DIFFERENT AGE GROUPS

AGE	BACTERIA	MOST EFFECTIVE ANTIBIOTICS
0-2 months	E. coli	Gentamicin
	Streptococcus group B	Penicillin
	Staphylococcus	Oxacillin
6 months-3 years	H. influenzae	Ampicillin, chloramphenicol
3-12 years	Pneumococcus	Penicillin
	Meningococcus	Penicillin

and *Escherichia coli*. The infection usually is acquired from the mother at birth during the baby's passage through the birth canal. Neonatal meningitis is particularly severe and dangerous, possibly because the infant's nervous system has yet to reach maturity and full development. Treatment consists of antibiotic therapy, the specific drugs being chosen on the basis of the microorganism found. The usual antibiotics used include ampicillin, kanamycin or gentamicin and often a combination of two of the above. The course of treatment extends for 3-4 weeks. Despite adequate antibiotic treatment, neonatal meningitis has a high mortality rate and a high incidence of long-term neurologic impairment in many of the survivors. Sequelae may include mental retardation, cerebral palsy and epilepsy; all are quite serious complications.

In infants and children from 6 months to 3 years of age, the most common agent causing bacterial meningitis is *Hemophilus influenzae*. This organism is also quite virulent and produces serious infections. The antibiotics of choice include ampicillin and/or chloramphenicol. The course of treatment usually is 10-14 days and depends on the response of the patient to treatment. Mortality, approximately 5%, is much lower than for neonatal meningitis; however, long-term sequelae may be present in 40-60% of patients with this disease. These problems may include fluid accumulation inside the brain (hydrocephalus), deafness, mental retardation, sensorimotor problems and epilepsy. Unfortunately, there is no way to prevent the sequelae in patients who have acquired this infection, but certainly early treatment is helpful in preventing some of the damage. However, even with prompt institution of therapy, major complications can occur.

H. influenzae can produce many types of infection, including ear infections, pneumonia and arthritis. It is not known why this organism invades the nervous system and produces meningitis in some children but not in others. Although this bacterium can be spread from one person to another by direct contact (touching, coughing or sneezing directly onto another person), the great majority of people who contract *H. influenzae* infection do not develop meningitis. It is not necessary to be overly alarmed if a child has been exposed to another child known to have *H. influenzae;* it is sufficient merely to observe the exposed child closely for any signs of illness, such as fever, irritability, headache or vomiting. If any of these symptoms develop, the child should be taken promptly to a physician for examination.

In older children, over the age of 3 years, two strains of bacteria seem to predominate in causing meningitis. These are *Diplococcus pneumoniae* and *Neisseria meningitidis*. Each of these organisms can be treated adequately with intravenous penicillin therapy. Meningitis produced by these bacteria can cause long-term sequelae but somewhat less frequently than those from organisms that have a predilection for younger children. Residual problems, especially after pneumococcal meningitis, can include deafness, blindness, epilepsy and psychomotor retardation. *Neisseria meningitidis* can cause a particularly rapid and fulminant generalized infection with shock, uncontrolled bleeding and death. With prompt recognition and treatment, however, the infection can be treated adequately.

No pattern of contagiousness has been determined for pneumococcal infections, and there is no need to quarantine patients or to be overly concerned about exposure. Family members living in the same household as a child with meningococcal meningitis should be examined by a physician and watched closely for signs of illness. Prophylactic antibiotic therapy with rifampin or sulfonamides may be given to people who have had close contact with the patient.

120 INFECTIONS OF THE CENTRAL NERVOUS SYSTEM

The bacterium that causes tuberculosis can also cause meningitis in any age group. This type of infection is particularly serious and is associated with significant mortality rates as well as long-term serious residual problems in survivors. Diagnosis is more difficult because the tuberculum bacillus is not always easily seen under the microscope and because the spinal fluid abnormalities are not always readily diagnostic for tuberculosis.

Tuberculous meningitis usually is found in the presence of tuberculosis elsewhere in the body; for example, in the lungs. Routine tuberculin tests on a yearly basis should be encouraged in all children as well as in adults, and any conversion of a tuberculin test from negative to positive should warrant careful examination by the physician, as well as a chest x-ray. Anyone exposed to a patient with tuberculosis should have a skin test.

Treatment of tuberculous meningitis consists of multiple drug therapy for 18 months or longer. Not all of this treatment must be given in the hospital, however. When the child recovers from the serious acute illness he may go home and take antibiotics orally for the remainder of the course.

Common neurologic sequelae of tuberculous meningitis include hydrocephalus, atrophy of part of the brain resulting in weakness of one side of the body, epilepsy and mental retardation.

VIRAL (ASEPTIC) MENINGITIS. — Some viruses have a definite predilection for invading the central nervous system and cause meningitis when the membranes surrounding the brain are infected. Viral infections typically do not result in purulent meningitis but instead in a relatively milder inflammation; for this reason, it is termed "aseptic" meningitis. Viruses can also infect the brain substance itself and produce encephalitis.

There is no specific treatment for most types of viral meningitis, and antibiotics are of no value. This type of infection tends to be self-limited in many cases and does not cause serious long-term complications. One of the notable exceptions is herpes encephalitis, which is a devastating and often fatal disease.

Diagnosis is based on examination of spinal fluid, which typically has fewer abnormalities than in bacterial meningitis. Sometimes it is not possible to differentiate viral from bacterial disease, especially early in the course; in these instances, antibiotic therapy should be initiated until bacterial infection can be excluded.

Long-term residual problems can occur after viral meningitis but are relatively infrequent compared with bacterial meningitis. These include hydrocephalus, epilepsy, mental retardation and motor deficits. At present there is no effective way to prevent occurrence of these complications.

Treatment is symptomatic; that is, medication can be used to reduce fever and to control headache and muscle pain.

FUNGAL MENINGITIS. — Another type of microorganism that can produce serious infection in humans is the fungus. Several types of fungal infections are relatively common in certain regions of the United States. These are coccidioidomycosis (valley fever) and cryptococcosis (torulosis). Fungi enter the body via the respiratory tract and invade the lungs. However, they do not always produce an obvious illness. From the lung, a fungal infection can spread to the nervous system and produce meningitis. Fungal infection of the nervous system tends to be more insidious than that caused by bacteria; symptoms may be nonspecific and the disease may evolve slowly over the course of several weeks. Initial symptoms may consist only of headache, low-grade fever and loss of appetite. Impairment of mental function may develop, with loss of concentration and decreased memory. As the disease progresses, seizures or coma may develop.

Diagnosis is based on finding evidence of fungal infection in the spinal fluid. Treatment consists of antifungal agents such as amphotericin B, administered intravenously, and, at times, directly into the spinal fluid (intrathecal administration) over a period of weeks and sometimes months, depending on the rapidity with which the fungus is eliminated by the medication. The treatment itself is not without problems. Amphotericin B is a relatively toxic agent and can be harmful to the kidney. Tests of kidney function must be performed frequently as long as the patient requires treatment.

Although the treatment of fungal meningitis is potentially harmful to the patient, the risk of treatment is outweighed by the severity of the infection. Untreated, fungal meningitis has a very high mortality rate.

ENCEPHALITIS

Encephalitis is an inflammatory condition involving the brain substance, usually secondary to viral invasion of the central nervous system. Numerous types of viruses are known to produce encephalitis. These include arboviruses (generally carried by mosquitoes), herpes simplex, mumps and lymphocytic choriomeningitis. Rabies, although less common, produces a severe encephalitis also. The clinical symptomatology associated with encephalitis has a wide range, from mild headache and fever to drowsiness and, in severe cases, coma and death. There is no specific treatment for most types of encephalitis, and patients receive primarily supportive and symptomatic care with intravenous fluids and medication to relieve headache and reduce temperature. Recently, an antiviral drug called adenosine arabinoside (Ara-A) has been found to be effective in treating adults with herpes encephalitis. Its efficacy in children with this disease has yet to be established.

A second type of response to viral invasion of the brain is postinfectious encephalitis. In this case, symptoms are slow and insidious and consist of progressive decrease in mentation (dementia), seizures and motor dysfunction, occurring over a period of weeks or months. The virus that originally produced the symptoms no longer may be detectable in the brain but presumably has led to some chemical alteration that causes progressive debilitation. At present there is no effective treatment for this postinfectious form of encephalitis, and many patients have a progressive downhill course.

BRAIN ABSCESS

This is a localized area of infection confined to one part of the brain, with accumulation of pus in an encapsulated area. It is similar to an abscess or a boil on the skin, but because of its location inside the brain it may have very serious consequences. Since an abscess grows within the enclosed cavity of the skull, it produces pressure on adjacent areas of the brain. Symptoms depend on the part of the brain involved; for example, if it is in the motor cortex, weakness would result. The brain around the abscess swells (becomes edematous) and increases the pressure inside the head, causing headache, lethargy, vomiting, blurring of vision or double vision.

Brain abscesses can result from local spread of infection from sinuses, nose, ears and mastoids (air cells behind the ears) and also from spread of infection elsewhere in the body via the blood stream. Children with cyanotic congenital heart disease, valvular heart disease (e.g., from rheumatic fever) and infections on the valves of the heart (bacterial endocarditis) are especially prone to develop brain abscesses. The recognition of an abscess can be difficult because such infections tend to be slowly progressive and at times indolent. Early symptoms may be vague and include headaches, low-grade fever and irritability or lethargy. A history of infection elsewhere in the body, especially with such problems as acute sinusitis, is helpful. A careful neurologic examination looking for localized deficits is important.

Many organisms can cause abscess formation. Bacteria are the usual infecting agents, and some species that do not grow well in air (anaerobic) can grow well inside an encapsulated abscess.

Treatment usually is multifaceted. Intravenous antibiotic therapy should be initiated immediately and be continued for weeks or months. Very often neurosurgical intervention is also required to drain the pus from the abscess and to relieve pressure.

Brain abscesses constitute a serious medical problem, but, with early recognition and effective treatment, the outcome can be good. Permanent damage can result if, for instance, pressure from the abscess on adjacent brain tissue is significant enough to cause death of cells in that area. The situation can become life-threatening if the abscess breaks open and spreads pus through the ventricular system of the brain.

In summary, infections of the nervous system constitute a serious childhood problem. They may cause permanent sequelae with varying degrees of brain damage and, less frequently, may cause death. Early diagnosis and prompt institution of treatment are essential to decrease mortality and morbidity from these diseases.

12

HYPERACTIVITY SYNDROMES

ALL NORMAL, HEALTHY CHILDREN are active, at times to the point of irritation when parents would like "peace and quiet." Hyperactivity has become a favorite diagnosis of parents and teachers when a child's behavior irritates them. But at what point does activity really exceed the normal? When is a child *truly* "hyperactive"?

Hyperactivity is defined rather vaguely as movement in excess of normal daily activity. This definition is not useful, since there is a wide range of normal activity. It is more helpful to define hyperactive behavior by its components; that is, excessive *nondirected* movement, with short attention span and inability to concentrate on one thing for any period of time. Truly hyperactive children are unable to complete tasks because of this. Thus, in assessing a child for this problem, there are several areas of questioning that may help to differentiate normal from abnormal behavior. Is the child able to sit through his favorite television shows? Does he sit through a meal without getting up? Can he sit still when playing with a favorite toy? Does he sleep through the night?

It has been estimated that as many as 10% of children between 5 and 12 years of age are hyperactive. However, because of rather vague criteria, an accurate estimate is quite difficult. The hyperactivity or hyperkinesia syndrome has been linked with another entity, minimal cerebral dysfunction (MCD). Children with MCD are said to have hyperactive behavior, short attention span, learning disabilities, poor motor coordination, easy distractibility and impulsiveness. The cause of MCD is thought in some cases to be some mild brain damage in early life; for example, from perinatal anoxia, encephalitis, meningitis or head trauma. However, in many patients, no identifiable cause can be found.

CAUSES OF HYPERACTIVE BEHAVIOR

Hyperactive behavior may be the result of a variety of underlying problems. Children with MCD may exhibit hyperactivity along with other symptoms of neurologic dysfunction. These children may also have poor gross and fine motor control and difficulty in learning. *Constitutional hyperactivity* is the term applied to children who are otherwise normal but who exhibit excessive motor activity. These children usually show signs of increased activity from infancy, requiring less sleep than the average child of the same age. There often is a family history of hyperactivity, and the syndrome is more common in males than in females. The increased activity in children with constitutional hyperactive behavior tends to normalize as the children enter the teenage years. The underlying cause of this type of hyperactivity is not known, but one hypothesis is that such children have an immature nervous system or a deficiency of a chemical neurotransmitter; the deficiency "corrects" itself as the child gets older.

Situational hyperactivity is an intermittent form of increased motor activity that some children exhibit when confronted with a stressful situation. Such children may have normal levels of activity most of the time but when confronted with a situation that is anxiety-producing, they tend to react with a significant increase in motor activity. Children with learning disabilities, for example, may find school a stressful situation and react with hyperactive behavior. Other children may suddenly become hyperactive when there is stress in the home; for example, parental discord.

Hyperactive behavior is relatively common in children with *mental retardation. Phenobarbital therapy* prescribed, for example, for control of seizures in children can produce hyperactive behavior as an unpleasant side effect. Other medications can also produce excessive increases in activity. These include prednisone, a steroid hormone used in the treatment of a variety of neuromuscular and dermatologic disorders, and chloral hydrate, a drug that usually is used as a sedative but that can produce just the opposite results in children. An abnormal increase in activity of the thyroid gland, hyperthyroidism, can also cause an increase in motor activity and should be considered in the differential diagnosis of a child with hyperactivity. It is also seen in children with chronic lead poisoning.

TREATMENT OF HYPERACTIVITY SYNDROME

Treatment of hyperactivity in childhood should be individualized depending on the reason for the abnormal behavior. A child with hyperthyroidism should have the thyroid condition remedied. When medication such as phenobarbital produces hyperactivity, this drug should be withdrawn and other medications, ones that are less likely to cause behavior problems, substituted. A child with situational hyperactivity will benefit most by modification of that part of his environment that is producing stress; for example, a child with learning difficulty should be placed in a classroom situation in which he will receive special assistance for his disability. Children who are responding adversely to parental strife may benefit from family counseling to remedy the underlying problem.

This leaves two large groups: those with constitutional hyperactivity and those with behavior associated with evidence of brain damage or mild neurologic dysfunction. It is not always necessary to treat children with constitutional hyperactive behavior; some do well developmentally and in school despite the relative increase in motor activity. Many children who have constitutional hyperactivity or MCD are, however, impeded in their ability to learn because of excessive movement and inability to concentrate for any length of time. These children deserve treatment to try to normalize activity.

Treatment should take a three-pronged approach: appropriate educational placement, psychiatric help or counseling and medication.

The goal of therapy is to bring the activity level to normal and to increase the child's ability to concentrate. Medications used in the treatment of hyperactivity are not meant to sedate the child; sedation merely replaces one form of abnormal behavior with another.

There are two general categories of drugs currently used in the treatment of hyperactive behavior: stimulants and antipsychotics.

Stimulant Medications

For many years it has been recognized that certain drugs that are stimulants in adults produce the opposite reaction in children. This is true of the *amphetamines*. Normal children may become apathetic and sedated when amphetamines are administered; hyperactive children tend to have their behavior approach a normal degree of activity. The reason for this paradoxical action is not clear. One hypothesis, as yet unproved, is that hyperactive children have a relative deficiency of certain chemicals that act as neurotransmitters in the brain; these deficiencies then presumably are remedied by administration of certain medications. Whatever the underlying mechanism, drugs in the amphetamine family are quite effective in treating many children with hyperactive behavior. The agent most frequently used is methylphenidate (Ritalin). This drug usually is given in two divided doses, once in the morning and again at noon. Methylphenidate may produce insomnia if administered later in the day. Usual dosage is 10–30 milligrams per day. It generally is unnecessary to exceed this dose, and if the child does not respond to this, another medication should be substituted. Methylphenidate is very effective in decreasing hyperactive and impulsive behavior and in improving concentration; however, some children, especially those with evidence of other neurologic dysfunction, may react adversely to this drug and it actually may increase the degree of motor activity.

Side effects of methylphenidate are rare, but, when present, may consist of a skin rash, loss of appetite, abdominal pain, insomnia or nervousness. If these occur, alteration of dosage or change to a different medication is advisable. Reports of impairment of linear growth (height) have been published recently, but other investigators have found no long-term alteration in height or other growth parameters in children taking methylphenidate.

Many physicians believe that methylphenidate should be given to the child only at times during which the hyperactive behavior would be most detrimental; for example, during school hours. They prescribe this medication for weekday use and suggest that the parents not administer it over the weekends and vacation periods. This is a sensible approach, since any side effects of medication would be somewhat minimized and yet the child would have the benefit of increased concentration and attention span at a time when he is learning.

Dextroamphetamine (Dexedrine) is another stimulant drug that sometimes is used to control hyperactive behavior. The daily dosage in this case usually is 5–15 milligrams, and again is most effectively administered in the morning before school. Side effects are similar to those produced by methylphenidate. There is no evidence that administration of the amphetamine drugs for hyperactivity results in physical or psychologic dependence on the drug or in drug addiction.

Pemoline (Cylert) is a drug that recently has been introduced for the control of hyperactive behavior. It appears to be useful in those children who have adverse reactions to methylphenidate. Dosage is 37–75 milligrams per day in a single morning dose; side effects may include skin rash and, rarely, damage to liver cells. Children on pemoline should have tests of liver function performed at periodic intervals. If signs of liver damage occur, the medication should be withdrawn.

Major Tranquilizers

Some hyperactive children, especially those who have signs of brain damage or mild neurologic dysfunction, may not respond to the stimulant medications. Often their behavior is also characterized as aggressive, impulsive and negative. In these patients, a group of drugs known as phenothiazines, generally used as antipsychotic agents, may be effective in altering behavior. The agent most commonly used is thioridazine (Mellaril), which is a relatively mild drug but which may result in striking improvement in symptoms. Thioridazine usually is administered in divided doses throughout the day, and the dosage range for children is 20–100 milligrams per day. Mild side effects of nausea and sleepiness may be seen; more serious side effects are rare but may include skin rash, depression of white blood cell count, liver damage and involuntary movements and postures (dystonia). The occurrence of any of the severe complications warrants prompt discontinuation of medication. Chlorpromazine (Thorazine) is another major tranquilizer occasionally used in children with the complex of symptoms described above. Chlorpromazine is more potent than thioridazine and requires close medical supervision during its use. This agent is also given in divided doses throughout the day, with a total daily dose of 10–30 milligrams. Mild side effects include drowsiness, dry mouth and, rarely, dizziness secondary to a decrease in blood pressure. More severe complications include depression of white blood cell count, skin rash, abnormal movements, dystonic posture and jaundice. Medication should be withdrawn if these occur.

Other medications are less frequently used for the control of hyperactive behavior. These include imipramine (Tofranil) and diphenhydramine (Benadryl). These drugs appear to be less effective than the amphetamines and phenothiazines but may benefit a limited number of children.

Any drug therapy must be individualized. Dosage must be balanced according to each child's response; if one medication does not appear to be effective in recommended therapeutic doses, another should be substituted rather than increasing the amount of the original drug to toxic levels. Similarly, duration of therapy must also be individualized. Many children no longer will need medication by the time they are 12 or 13; others will require continued management well into adolescence. The care of these children is best handled by a physician familiar with the symptoms, medications used and side effects.

ALTERNATIVE APPROACHES TO THERAPY

Other approaches to the treatment of the hyperactive child have been suggested but their effectiveness is unproved as

Alternative Approaches to Therapy

yet. These include behavior modification, a special diet free from food additives and salicylates and megavitamin therapy.

Advocates of *behavior modification* suggest that hyperactivity is a learned behavior pattern that is unwittingly reinforced through words or actions by the parents. Therapy centers around teaching the parents how to positively reinforce (reward) good behavior while negatively reinforcing unpleasant behavior. It certainly is true that some parents reinforce their child's negative behavior, for example, by laughing at a child who has just used a "bad" word for the first time. However, it may be somewhat simplistic to view all hyperactive children as being products of their environment without taking into account other possible causes; for example, brain damage and lead poisoning. No large studies have been published as yet that confirm or deny the effectiveness of behavior modification, and this form of treatment may be useful in a select group of children.

Diet therapy has received much publicity recently. One popular diet is based on the exclusion of all food additives and salicylates from the diet. Improvement in activity levels has been reported in some children on this diet, although other studies have not been able so far to demonstrate a significant response in large numbers of children. It may be worthwhile to try this form of treatment although the diet is quite restrictive and requires a significant amount of time spent in food shopping and preparation. The parents must be aware of this and be willing to carry out the program. A dietitian should be involved to ensure that the diet is well balanced and provides all essential vitamins, minerals, etc.

Megavitamin therapy involves treatment with very large doses of vitamins, especially those of the B complex. The theory behind such treatment is that children with hyperactivity have a chemical abnormality that is correctable with high doses of vitamins. However, this is purely speculative and there is no evidence that megavitamin therapy improves hyperactive behavior in any consistent way.

Finally, it has been suggested that the caffeine in coffee may improve hyperactivity. Again, no consistent benefits have been observed in most children given this mode of therapy.

Coffee can produce stomach upset and bladder irritation, so it is unwise to suggest this as a treatment unless controlled studies demonstrate real effectiveness.

PROGNOSIS

It is difficult to determine the long-term outlook for a child with hyperactive behavior, since the problem may have any one of numerous diverse causes. It is fair to say that children with hyperactivity alone have a good possibility of doing quite well as adults. The behavior problem tends to come under control during adolescence, medications no longer are required and the person can lead a normal life. Obviously, if the hyperactivity is associated with mental retardation or brain damage, the prognosis is more guarded and depends on the extent of the underlying problem.

13

LEARNING DISABILITIES

PROBABLY no topic is receiving more publicity and interest within the educational system today than that of learning disabilities. It is an area that is not fully understood but about which many theories are being offered. This discussion will deal with general concepts of learning disabilities, with emphasis on recognition and possibilities for treatment.

DEFINITION OF LEARNING DISABILITIES

Many people are not clear about what learning disabilities mean. Children with learning disorders have *normal* intelligence but have isolated difficulty in one or more school-related areas. It is very important to emphasize the normal IQ in this group, since the parents especially are concerned about their child being retarded if he seems unable to learn. In children with multiple learning disabilities, sometimes it is difficult to establish normal intelligence, but this usually can be accomplished by thorough neurologic and psychometric evaluations. Children with mental retardation are delayed in all aspects of developmental functions; for example, comprehension, visual motor skills, vocabulary and gross and fine motor function. Children with learning disabilities function at a normal to above-normal developmental level in some areas but are behind in others. This is reflected in standard tests of intelligence such as the Wechsler Intelligence Scale for Children (WISC), in which there may be a wide spread between verbal and performance IQ in children with learning disabilities. Spurious test results can be obtained in a child with poor concentrating ability or short attention span, and these problems should be carefully noted in a child whose performance on such tests is lower than expected.

CAUSES OF LEARNING DISABILITIES

No single underlying cause has been identified in children with learning disorders. There is a hereditary predilection for a specific type of reading dysfunction that predominates in males who are otherwise totally normal. This probably accounts for only a small percentage of children with learning problems. Many children who are evaluated for learning disorders have a history of perinatal difficulties, including prematurity, breech delivery, umbilical cord wrapped around the neck, etc. A causal relationship between perinatal difficulties and learning disorders is difficult to prove, however. Other children have a history of encephalitis or meningitis. Again, the causal relationship is not clear but certainly suggestive, since these infections do invade the nervous system and can result in residual brain damage.

Finally, there is a rare developmental abnormality involving dysfunction of the dominant (usually left) parietal lobe of the brain, resulting in the Gerstmann syndrome. This is a well-defined abnormality consisting of four components: finger agnosia (lack of ability to identify individual fingers), right-left disorientation, dysgraphia (inability to write) and dyscalculia (inability to do math).

IDENTIFICATION OF THE CHILD WITH POTENTIAL LEARNING DISABILITIES

Any child who is not performing at grade level is suspect for learning disabilities. The original legal definition of a learning-disabled child is one who is 2 years behind grade level in one or more areas, but this is an arbitrary criterion that serves only to delay identification of such children in many instances. Several problems must be sorted out from learning disabilities. Lack of motivation on the part of the child certainly can produce learning problems. Poor motivation may be due to lack of stimulation at home, family discord, poor self-image, childhood depression or a feeling of ostracism (for example, a child from a minority group in a classroom in which teacher and other students are of different ethnic or socioeconomic backgrounds). Hyperactive behavior with associated difficulty in concentrating and short attention span can also interfere with learning. Unsuspected hearing and visual deficits sometimes can present with difficulty in learning. Unrealistic expectations on the part of parents and sometimes teachers can lead to a suspicion that a child has learning disabilities. All of these possibilities should be considered and explored before a child is labeled as learning disabled.

The potential for learning difficulties may be suspected as early as kindergarten; for example, in a child who has poor drawing skills or who has significant difficulty in learning the alphabet. However, it is more common to have such children identified in the first or second grade, after they have demonstrated marked delays in acquisition of math or reading skills.

There are several approaches to evaluation of a child with suspected learning disabilities. Many school districts coordinate the evaluation within the school. Typically, these children are given intelligence and achievement tests by the school psychologist; they may have a speech and language evaluation by a speech therapist employed by the schools; they then may be referred to a pediatrician or pediatric neurologist, where one is available, to "rule out neurologic problems." This is an extremely misleading concept that appears to be widespread in educational circles. Although the neural mechanisms by which learning occurs are poorly understood, it is clear that normal acquisition of knowledge requires an intact nervous system; thus, any child with learning disabilities has, in effect, a "neurologic problem." The real question should be: Does the child have a specific, identifiable neurologic disorder that might require medical treatment (for example, seizure disorder, brain tumor, etc.)? A very small number of children diagnosed as learning disabled do turn out to have neurologic disorders; Duchenne's muscular dystrophy, adrenoleukodystrophy, hydrocephalus, Arnold-Chiari malformation and petit mal epilepsy are a few of the diagnoses that have been identified during the course of evaluating children for "learning disabilities."

The medical approach to learning disabilities should be comprehensive and include a team of professionals who have expertise in the field of learning problems. At the University Hospital Medical Center in San Diego, a learning evaluation clinic (LEC) was instituted to comprehensively evaluate children referred for suspected learning problems. Members of the LEC team include a pediatric neurologist, speech pathologist, occupational therapist, visual motor therapist and social worker. Ancillary facilities within the hospital are available for audiology, psychometric testing, psychiatric therapy and dietary management, if the team believes that any of these are indicated.

Each member of the team performs a diagnostic evaluation on each patient. Parents are interviewed in depth by the social worker, who also contacts the schoolteacher and psychologist for their impressions. The group then gathers for a staff meeting, during which each member's findings are discussed and a diagnostic and treatment plan are designed. A report then is made to the parents and the school with suggestions for educational and remedial approaches. Sometimes additional treatment by a speech or occupational therapist is suggested.

A routine electroencephalogram has little value in the evaluation of a child with learning disabilities. If the physician believes that there is a possibility of an undiagnosed seizure disorder or other evidence of specific neurologic disease, an EEG may be in order; for children with no abnormality other than difficulty in learning, an EEG probably is a waste of money and time on the part of the parents.

A neurologic evaluation to screen for learning disabilities typically includes those items outlined in Chapter 2: a complete neurologic examination, tests of hearing and visual acuity, a Denver Developmental Screening Test in younger children, a design copying test, draw-a-person test, grade-appropriate tests of reading, writing, math and spelling and some assessment of language and auditory skills.

TYPES OF LEARNING DISABILITIES

The problem of learning disabilities is a continuum and sometimes it is difficult to place the child in a clear diagnostic category. General groups can at least be defined, although it should be remembered that few children have isolated deficits. General categories include:

Dyslexia—isolated inability to read.
Dyscalculia—inability to calculate or do math problems.
Dysgraphia—inability to write.
Receptive aphasia—inability to comprehend spoken language.
Expressive aphasia—inability to express oneself verbally, even though comprehension is intact.
Gerstmann syndrome—complex of dyscalculia, dysgraphia, finger agnosia and right-left disorientation.

UNDERLYING PROBLEMS ASSOCIATED WITH LEARNING DISABILITIES

Learning to read is a complex skill that brings into play many facets of the nervous system. These are taken for granted by the average person because they are integrated at a subconscious level, and so it is difficult for most people to understand how a child with normal intelligence can be unable to learn to read. In order to understand why children have learning disabilities, it is helpful to break down specific learned skills into their component parts. The ability to read, for example, requires that the person have intact function in the following areas: sound-symbol associations, that is, what sound is associated with the letter "b"; word-symbol associations, that is, what symbol is associated with the word "cat"; sound blending, that is, putting together the sound of individual letters to form a word; auditory discrimination, to tell one letter sound from another; visual memory, to remember what words have come before; visual tracking, to follow words smoothly across the page; right-left orientation, since the eyes must move first from left to right, then down and back to the left, and so on. In reading aloud, visual-oral coordination is required as well.

It is clear from the above illustrations that reading is an extremely complex process, and inability to perform any one of the above maneuvers can result in a form of learning dysfunction.

A similar problem exists for mathematics. In order to add 28 plus 35, the child must have a concept of what numbers mean; be able to retain in memory the sum of 8 plus 5; know right from left, since he must begin adding the right-hand column of numbers and then carry the 1 to the left; and be able to coordinate eye and hand to write the numbers (visual motor coordination).

In writing, other skills come into play. Adequate fine motor coordination is necessary to hold the pencil and guide it along the paper to form legible symbols; visual motor skills are also necessary to form legible symbols. Ability to cross midline is necessary, that is, a right-handed child must be able to coordinate his hand when writing on the left side of the page; right-left orientation is important for writing comprehensible sentences. Spatial orientation must be intact to prevent letter reversal.

When learned skills are analyzed in this way, it is clearly not enough to say that a child cannot read; rather, it is necessary to determine wherever possible the specific reason for the child's inability to read, so that therapy can be aimed at that problem.

MANAGEMENT OF THE CHILD WITH LEARNING DISABILITIES

There are several schools of thought as to the best educational or therapeutic approach to the child with learning disabilities. One is to teach to the child's strengths, that is, concentrate on the skills he does have and minimize his weaknesses. In this way he is taught to avoid areas in which he does not do well, while at the same time being allowed to excel at those tasks that are easy for him. This approach has its benefits because the child achieves self-esteem by doing well in certain facets of learning. Theoretically, this approach could be detrimental in the long run. A child who cannot read, for example, may be able to learn well using audiovisual aids (tape recorder, educational TV, and others). Modern-day civilization is complex, however. If we buy clothes, we must read the labels to find out how they are to be cleaned. To put together a child's train set we must be able to read instructions.

In adult life, the person with dyslexia will be limited by an inability to read directions on items bought in the store, to follow road maps or to read the newspaper. He may even have difficulty in filling out a job application because he is unable to read the questions. Thus, it is somewhat compelling to try to treat the underlying problem while the person is young, if he is to have the best chance of leading a fully normal life in today's world.

A second approach is to teach to the child's weakness, concentrating on all the problem areas. The difficulty with this is that children with normal intelligence realize that they are unable to successfully master a subject that other children can; they may get easily frustrated by constant reminders of their disability. It is best to combine the two approaches. The child should be encouraged to master material he *can* do and receive positive reinforcement in the form of verbal praise and good grades for this, while at the same time working on those areas in which he has difficulty.

Specific approaches to the problem generally are of two types. The first approach is within the school. Most schools now have teachers specially trained in learning disabilities. Some children go to regular classes most of the day, with the exception of a period of time spent with a learning resources teacher concentrating on problem areas. Other children with multiple learning disabilities may need to be in a special class exclusively, since they require full-time concentration on their learning difficulties. The choice of classes depends on the extent of the problem; the child with isolated dyslexia or dyscalculia is best placed in a regular class and taken out only for reading or math whereas a child with severe difficulty in reading, writing *and* math may benefit best from continued assistance in a self-contained classroom.

The second approach to treatment involves an attack on the underlying problem by outside specialists. A child with right-left confusion or spatial disorientation, poor fine motor or visual motor skills may receive treatment by an occupational therapist in the form of sensory integration exercises. That is, using simultaneous verbal and tactile stimulation, the child is taught to distinguish right from left, up from down, etc. Similar therapeutic approaches are taken by speech therapists for children with auditory perceptual problems and language disabilities. It has been debated whether this form of therapy generalizes and carries over to improve school performance. The answer still is not clear, since it is difficult to do controlled studies. Perhaps the individual attention alone is enough to increase a child's self-image and in that way improve school performance. Although the effectiveness of these approaches has not been fully substantiated as yet, it makes sense, based on the underlying problems that give rise to learning disabilities, to try them, especially since there is no proved effective alternative.

Other methods that are advocated by certain groups have little proved value and may be costly for the parent. These include visual training to exercise eye muscles, patterning exercises in which the child relearns to crawl, etc., and special diets.

SPECIAL PROBLEMS OF THE LEARNING-DISABLED CHILD

Adults sometimes underestimate a child's awareness and insight. Children with learning disabilities are acutely aware that there is something "different" about them. They realize that they are unable to master certain skills that other children find easy. If children are not recognized as having learning disabilities, they eventually become frustrated at their shortcomings. They may begin to "act out" in class and may become behavior problems. It has been estimated that as many as 95% of children referred to a child psychiatrist for behavior problems have learning disabilities. It should be recognized that many of these behavior problems are secondary to frustration. Such children are not "bad" and should not be treated as such. Early recognition of their learning difficulties and subsequent appropriate classroom placement or institution of therapy may avert later behavior problems.

14

SPEECH AND LANGUAGE DISORDERS

THE ABILITY to communicate verbally is a highly sophisticated function. Inability to understand or to effectively express oneself with language can be a severe detriment to normal learning. There are two major areas in which deficits may occur: impairment of speech itself, making attempts at communication ineffective, and disorders of language comprehension or expression. Under these major categories there are numerous subgroups of problems. These will be discussed in this chapter.

NORMAL SPEECH AND LANGUAGE DEVELOPMENT

The earliest form of vocalization that an infant makes is a reflexive cry, which is present from birth. By 2 months of age, this cry undergoes some differentiation, and one quality of cry will be used to indicate hunger, another pain and yet another the desire to be held. Mothers usually can differentiate these various appeals. By 3–4 months of age, the infant begins to vocalize in another way, by cooing, consisting primarily of vowel sounds, and by gurgling and squealing. He also begins to laugh out loud at about this time.

By 6 months of age, the infant usually has developed babbling, which consists of both vowel and consonant utterances. Within the next 2 months he begins to have repetitive utterances, for example, da-da, ga-ga and, at times, to use these with inflections that indicate that he wants something. At this age, these vocalizations have no specific meaning to the infant, so that he does not identify "da-da" with his father. By

9–10 months, the infant begins to imitate words spoken to him; for example, ma-ma, bye-bye. He also begins to imitate movements associated with certain words; for instance, waving his hand while saying bye-bye. At this stage, the infant also learns the meanings of certain words; when asked "Where is your doll?" he may look at his doll.

By the end of the first year of life, most children have acquired the ability to use one or two words in a relatively meaningful fashion. These words most often are "ma-ma" and "da-da." Comprehension of words exceeds the ability to speak at this point; a 1-year-old may be able to point to his nose when asked, even though he may not say the word.

In the next 12 months, spoken vocabulary and comprehension of words increase tremendously. Some children may not have intelligible speech before 18 months of age, although they are prolific at babbling. By 2 years, however, children should have a vocabulary of 100–300 words and are able to name most of the familiar people and objects in their environment. At this age, the average child can put two words together to form a simple sentence; for example, "go bye-bye," "want cookie," etc. Expressive language also consists of noun, verb and some pronoun usage. Receptively, the youngster can listen to short stories, respond to simple picture pointing tasks and carry out simple commands. Approximately 50% of the 2-year-old's speech is intelligible to us.

Speech no longer is purely imitative by this age. The child begins to generalize from his experience with communication and to experiment with new phrases. For example, he may have learned from parents to say "more milk" but now may experiment with a new combination of words, "more cookies," to get what he wants. He thus has entered the stage of *creative* speech.

Between the ages of 2 and 3, the child's ability to communicate increases greatly. New vocabulary is accumulated almost daily. The child now expects others to *listen* to him when he speaks, demonstrating an awareness of language as a form of communication. At this age he uses more nouns, pronouns, verbs, prepositions and conjunctions. Awareness of syntax, that is, grammatical order of words in a sentence, becomes apparent at this age also. By 3 years of age, the average child can put at least three words together to form a sentence and uses the pronoun "I" correctly (e.g., "I want a cookie"). At least 80% of speech should be intelligible to the listener by this time. Pronunciation of certain phonemes (articulation of letter sounds) may not be completely achieved as yet, and the child may lisp (thun for sun) or substitute w for r (wabbit for rabbit).

The 4-year-old child has effectively dealt with this problem and now has a relatively mature language. Pronunciation of phonemes is good but still may be variable for the next 3–4 years. Vocabulary is large and the child can carry on a conversation easily and with some individual style. He should be intelligible to listeners virtually 100% of the time. Receptively, he comprehends meanings of such prepositions as behind, beside, under; he can follow a 2-stage command and recalls a nonsense syllable after a 30-second delay.

By the age of 5, speech should be close to adult levels in terms of syntax and intelligibility. At this age, children can distinguish with accuracy between two similar phonemes (for example, "k" and "t") repeated to them, even though they still may have difficulty in controlling oral musculature consistently enough to pronounce the phonemes correctly themselves. Oral blending of two consonants ("pr," "bl") usually is established between the ages of 5 and 6. Phonemic control should be good by the age of 7 or 8. Between 5 and 6 years of age, the average child will have acquired enough language skills so that he is ready to learn to read. Comprehension consists of basic concept understanding, e.g., center, middle, last; following a 3-stage command; and recalling a nonsense syllable after a 40–45-second latency.

DISORDERS OF SPEECH PRODUCTION

Speech production requires the presence of certain senses and skills. The individual must be able to hear, process and perceive normal voice frequencies in order to reproduce sounds accurately. He must have normal strength and coordination of tongue, lips, pharynx, larynx and facial muscles. He must have cortical control over these muscles in order to voluntarily place the oral muscles in proper position to articulate a certain sound. He must be able to perceive differences in sounds (auditory perception) and must be able to integrate sounds centrally in order to comprehend what they mean (sound-symbol associations) and to express his thoughts verbally.

Production of speech may be inhibited in several ways. A child who cannot perceive sounds will be unable to produce speech that is normal in volume, inflection and pronunciation. A normal infant who is placed in an environment devoid of verbal stimulation may have paucity of speech because there was no role model from which to learn. A child who has been the subject of physical or emotional abuse may not speak in an effort to keep from being hurt further. Autistic children characteristically have little speech for reasons that are not clear (the mechanisms underlying infantile autism are not known).

The mechanics of faulty speech production in children without the above problems usually are related to impairment of voluntary control over oral musculature. *Dysarthria* is the term used to describe unclear speech production associated with deficits in respiration, phonation, articulation and prosody. Dysarthria can result from damage to any of several areas of the brain, and the quality of the dysarthric speech usually will reflect the impairment of a particular part of the brain.

Pseudobulbar speech is the result of bilateral cortical damage. This damage impairs the normal function of the upper motor neurons (see Chap. 10) in the cortex, which normally control muscle strength and coordination, and produces a spastic dysarthria because of disinhibition of the lower motor neurons, which control facial and oral muscles. (These lower motor neurons are located in the brainstem and originate in the cranial nerve nuclei.)

A child with pseudobulbar paralysis may have some or all of the following abnormalities on physical examination: a hyperactive gag reflex; uncoordinated movements of the tongue and a persistent tongue thrust (an involuntary thrusting forward of the tongue on any tactile stimulation); uncoordinated lip

Disorders of Speech Production

opening and closure; persistent and excessive drooling; weakness of facial muscles; hoarseness; and a hypernasal sound to the voice due to decreased and uncoordinated palatal movements.

Pseudobulbar speech is typically strained, hypernasal and irregular in quality and words are slurred and may be unintelligible. Voice often reflects lack of proper intonation, loudness and rate. Children with pseudobulbar palsy may have difficulty with feeding from early infancy because of poor coordination of the tongue in moving food to the back of the mouth and because of the hyperactive gag reflex, which produces choking and gagging whenever food touches the palate. These infants tend to have excessive and persistent drooling and speech usually is delayed.

Bulbar paralysis occurs as a result of damage to the brainstem and cranial nerve nuclei and produces a lower motor neuron lesion with decreased gag reflex, poor palatal elevation and flaccid weakness of the oral and pharyngeal muscles. A flaccid dysarthria usually results, in which speech is slurred and hypernasal. Bulbar speech may result from tumors or infections involving the brainstem or from myasthenia gravis when oral and pharyngeal muscles are involved. At times, a palatal lift, fitted by an orthodontist, can decrease the nasal quality of the speech by elevating the palate.

Damage to the cerebellum may also produce an abnormality of speech called ataxic speech. This typically consists of loss of normal rhythm of speech; words are spoken in a slow, monotonous manner and speech is irregular, jerky and explosive. This type of problem can occur after anoxic damage to the cerebellum, certain infectious diseases (e.g., acute cerebellar ataxia) and tumors involving the cerebellum.

Stuttering is a disorder of speech that consists of difficulty in moving from one phoneme to the next, with explosive repetition or prolongation of certain phonemes. Stuttering typically begins between the ages of 3 and 4, and in males more often than in females. In many children who develop this problem it is transient. However, some continue to stutter indefinitely. Physicians and speech pathologists differ in their opinions as to the etiology of stuttering; some adhere to a physical basis whereas others attribute dysfluency to emotional causations. The most effective modes of therapy usually combine some direct work with the stuttering in addition to psychologic counseling.

DISORDERS OF LANGUAGE

Speech is the mechanical means by which we *communicate*. The ability to *communicate* with one another depends on intact *language*. Verbal and written communication require a complex series of integrative functions. Loss of any one of the steps involved in comprehension or expression of language can result in inability to communicate and thus learn with meaning.

AUDITORY PERCEPTUAL PROBLEMS

Comprehension of verbal or written language depends first on intact perception. It is important not to confuse "acuity" with perception, since the majority of youngsters suffering from perceptual disorders manifest good peripheral hearing. The primary sensory function, vision or hearing, must be intact. After the stimulus (set of words) is received, it must be *identified* and a meaning attached to it; it must be *discriminated* from other sets of words; it must be retained in sequential memory; it must be *compared* with other sets of words in order to comprehend and retrieve significant acts of language.

Testing for Auditory Perceptual Problems

Auditory retention can be tested by having the child repeat a sentence or a series of numbers forward and backward after the examiner. The norms for various ages are listed in Table 14–1.

Auditory discrimination is the ability to detect differences between either linguistic or nonlinguistic sounds. This can be evaluated by presenting the child with two sounds (ch-sh) and asking if they are the same or different. By the age of 7, dis-

TABLE 14-1.—AUDITORY RETENTION SKILLS IN CHILDHOOD

AGE IN YEARS	NUMBERS FORWARD	NUMBERS BACKWARD	MEMORY FOR WORDS IN SENTENCES
2½–3	2	—	2–3
3–4	3	—	4–6
4½–5	4	—	7–10
6	6	—	10–14
7	6–7	3	16
9	7	4	16
12	7	5	16

crimination of similar but different sounds should be relatively intact.

Knowledge of concepts should also be tested. Between the ages of 5 and 7, for example, most children (given a home environment in which communication is good) can tell the difference between big and small, before and after, up and down, same and different. These are basic concepts that are important foundations to learning and to communication.

Knowledge of receptive vocabulary skills can be evaluated by several methods. The child can be given a word and asked to point to the appropriate picture from a page containing several different drawings. He can also be given a word and asked to explain what it means (for example, "What is a lamp?"). Or he can be given a sentence and asked to fill in the missing word (for example, "The last car of a train is called a———").

The ability to sequence sounds is an important function that can be tested in the following way. A series of different sounds may be presented to the child and he is asked to repeat them (e.g., puh-tuh-kuh). Repetition of words in a sentence or of a series of numbers will also test for sequencing ability, as will repetition of the alphabet in the school-age child.

If any of the above tests is not performed adequately, the child should be referred to a speech pathologist, who can do more thorough testing and design a program of speech and/or language therapy that will concentrate on treating the communication problem.

DEVELOPMENTAL APHASIA

The term *aphasia* literally means "without speech." It usually is applied to adults who have lost the ability to comprehend language (receptive aphasia) or to express what they want to say (expressive aphasia) because of damage to speech centers in the brain. (The dichotomy of receptive-expressive aphasia seldom exists within an aphasic population.) Some children, however, are delayed in acquiring speech because of a developmental aphasia, presumably due to some early damage to speech centers. The diagnosis of developmental aphasia must be reserved for children who are not deaf, who are not mentally retarded and who are not autistic, since these three factors may also result in delayed speech acquisition.

Children with receptive aphasia are unable to formulate a meaning for words; that is, they cannot acquire symbols for a language system. The word "cat," for instance, cannot be associated with the household pet. If the child cannot make sense of words he hears, his own language will be impaired also, since he cannot express himself in words that have no meaning for him. Impairment in basic perceptual processes also contributes to aphasia syndromes.

Children with developmental aphasia usually present with severely delayed language. It often is difficult to document normal intelligence in such children. Standard tests of intelligence such as the WISC are unreliable because they depend on the child's ability to understand verbal instructions. A nonverbal assessment, such as the Leiter International Performance Scale, is a better test of ability in such children. Assessment of gross, fine and visual motor skills is also helpful, since many children with specific aphasia will have age-appropriate skills in other developmental spheres.

Aphasic children may get easily frustrated because of their inability to understand what is going on around them. They may have temper tantrums or destructive or hyperactive behavior. The possibility of developmental aphasia should be considered in a nonverbal child with behavior problems.

Often aphasic children will develop some rudimentary or automatic language skills. This does not rule out the possibility of an aphasic problem. The aphasic youngster may present a myriad of difficulties that run a continuum from no speech to impairment of basic concept comprehension.

Some children are able to comprehend speech but cannot express what they want to say. This problem is known as expressive or motor aphasia. Such children have a paucity of spoken vocabulary but are able to follow commands and comprehend the meaning of spoken language. Parents often relate that the child does not speak but points to something when he wants it. The evaluation of a child with suspected motor aphasia includes tests that do not require a verbal response. The Peabody Picture Vocabulary Test provides a set of pictures for the child to study. The examiner gives the child a word and asks him to point to the appropriate picture. A receptive vocabulary assessment can be performed in this way. Several other tests are available that examine receptive and expressive skills. These include the Picture Speech Discrimination Test and the Northwestern Syntax Screening Test.

Most children with aphasia have no specifically definable cause for the problem. Presumably it is the result of either a developmental anomaly of the nervous system or some early damage to the brain. However, there are a few cases in which a specific cause is found. Brain tumors, abscesses and arteriovenous malformations of the dominant hemisphere can result in aphasia secondary to compression or destruction of underlying brain tissue. Some children with epilepsy may have aphasia because of continuous epileptiform electrical discharges in the speech area of the brain. This condition is called *acquired epileptic aphasia*. Diagnosis can be made by the history of a child with seizures, who has stopped speaking after some speech acquisition had occurred. The electroencephalogram in such patients demonstrates epileptiform discharges over the left side of the brain. Treatment with anticonvulsant medications will, in some cases, improve speech development.

Awareness of the possibility of aphasia in a child with delayed speech acquisition is most important. These children should be referred to a competent speech pathologist for thorough evaluation and treatment and to a pediatric neurologist to rule out the possibility of a treatable problem such as acquired epileptic aphasia.

SELECTED BIBLIOGRAPHY

Berry, M. F.: *Language Disorders of Children* (New York: Appleton-Century-Crofts, 1969).

Eisenson, J.: *Aphasia in Children* (New York: Harper & Row, 1972).

Lowrey, G. H.: *Growth and Development of Children* (7th ed.; Chicago: Year Book Medical Publishers, Inc., 1978).

Menkes, J. H.: *Textbook of Child Neurology* (Philadelphia: Lea & Febiger, 1974).

Millichap, J. G.: *The Hyperactive Child with Minimal Brain Dysfunction* (Chicago: Year Book Medical Publishers, Inc., 1975).

Millichap, J. G. (ed.): *Learning Disabilities and Related Disorders: Facts and Currents Issues* (Chicago: Year Book Medical Publishers, Inc., 1977).

Mykelbust, H. R. (ed.): *Progress in Learning Disabilities* (New York: Grune & Stratton, 1968), Vol. 1.

Swaiman, K. F., and Wright, F. S.: Neurologic Disease Due to Developmental and Metabolic Defects, in Baker, A. B., and Baker, L. H. (eds.): *Clinical Neurology* (Hagerstown, Md.: Harper & Row, 1977), Vol. 3, Chap. 40.

Index

A

Abscess, brain, 116
　discussion of, 122-124
Acetazolamide: in seizures, 30
Acetylcholine, 108-109
Acidemia
　isovaleric, 78
　propionic, 78
Acrocephaly, 48
ACTH: in seizures, 30
Adenosine arabinoside: in encephalitis, 122
Adrenocorticotropic hormone: in seizures, 30
Adrenoleukodystrophy, 87
Adversive seizures, 24
Agenesis
　cerebellar, 46
　sacral, 52-54
Akinetic seizures, 23
Alleles, 70
Alpers' syndrome, 85-86
ALS, 105-106
Amino acid metabolism: inborn errors of, 75-77
Amniocentesis, 72
Amphetamines: in hyperactivity syndromes, 128-129
Amphotericin B: in fungal meningitis, 121
Amyotrophic lateral sclerosis, 105-106
Anencephaly, 5
Aneurysms, 55
Anomalies
　(See also Malformations)
　spinal cord, 49-54
Anterior horn cell
　definition of, 104
　diseases, 104-106

Anticonvulsants
　in cerebral palsy, 98
　in migraines, 35
　in seizures, 28
Aphasia
　definition of, 148
　developmental, 148-150
　epileptic, acquired, 149
　expressive, 137
　receptive, 137
Aqueductal stenosis, 43
Ara-A: in encephalitis, 122
Arachnoid villi, 43
Arnold-Chiari malformation, 47-48
Arteriography, 55
Arteriovenous malformation, 54
Aseptic meningitis, 120-121
Ataxia
　definition of, 92
　Friedreich's, 89
Ataxic speech, 145
Atonic diplegia, 95
Atrophy (see Muscle, atrophy)
Auditory perceptual problems, 146-147
　testing for, 146-147
Auditory retention skills: in childhood, 147
Autonomic nervous system: evaluation of, 16
Autosomal traits, 70
Axons, 106

B

Babinski sign, 14
Bacterial meningitis, 117-120
　types of, 118
Basal ganglia: degenerative diseases of, 88

Behavior
  hyperactive
    (*See also* Hyperactivity)
    causes of, 126–127
    modification in hyperactivity, 131
Benadryl: in hyperactive behavior, 130
Botulism, 109
Brain
  abscess, 116
    discussion of, 122–124
  anatomy of, 1, 2
  hemiatrophy of, 46
  tumors
    CT scan in, 57
    discussion of, 55–57
    headache due to, 39–40
Bruits, 17, 54
Bulbar palsy, 112

C

Café au lait spots: in neurofibromatosis, 73
Caffeine: in coffee, in hyperactivity syndromes, 131–132
Calcifications: intracranial, in Sturge-Weber syndrome, 61, 62
Carbamazepine: in seizures, 29–30
Carbohydrate metabolism: disorders of, 78–80
Central nervous system: infections of, 116–124
Cerebellar agenesis, 46
Cerebellar malformations, 46–48
Cerebral dominance: evaluation of, 15
Cerebral infarction, 45
Cerebral malformations, 42–46
Cerebral palsy, 90–102
  choreoathetoid, 91–92, 97–98
  diagnosis of, 92
  discussion of term, 90
  infant, head control in, 17
  orthopedic devices in, 99–101
  patterns of weakness in, 91
  prognosis in, 102
  surgery in, 101
  therapy in, 98–99
    rehabilitative, 99
Chairs: for cerebral palsy victims, 100, 101
Charcot-Marie-Tooth disease, 89
Chlorpromazine: in hyperactivity syndromes, 130
Chorea: Huntington's, 88
Choreoathetoid cerebral palsy, 91–92, 97–98
Chromosomes, 70–72
Clonazepam: in seizures, 30
Clonopin: in seizures, 30
Cluster headaches, 36–37
CNS: infections of, 116–124
Computerized tomography (*see* CT scan)
Congenital causes: of mental retardation, 62–63
Conus medullaris, 49
Convulsions, benign febrile, 24–25
  characteristics of, 25
Coordination tests, 15
Cranial nerves: evaluation of, 13, 14
Craniosynostosis, 48
Cranium, 2
CT scan
  in Arnold-Chiari malformation, 47
  in brain tumor, 57
  in hydrocephalus, 44
  in intracranial hemorrhage, 56
  in neurologic examination, 19
  in porencephaly, 46

INDEX

Cylert: in hyperactivity syndromes, 129

D

Dandy-Walker syndrome, 46–47
Dantrium: in cerebral palsy, 99
Dantrolene: in cerebral palsy, 99
Degenerative diseases
 of basal ganglia, 88
 of gray matter, 85–87
 of nervous system, 85–89
 of white matter, 87
Depression headaches, 38
Design copying skills: age achieved at, 10
Development (*see* Neurologic development)
Developmental aphasia, 148–150
Developmental reflexes: testing of, 16–17
Dexedrine: in hyperactivity syndromes, 129
Dextroamphetamine: in hyperactivity syndromes, 129
Diabetes mellitus, 82–84
 mental retardation due to, 64–65
Diamox: in seizures, 30
Diazepam: in cerebral palsy, 98–99
Diet therapy: in hyperactivity syndromes, 131
Dilantin: in seizures, 28–29
Diphenhydramine: in hyperactive behavior, 130
Diphenylhydantoin: in seizures, 28–29
Diplegia
 atonic, 95
 spastic, 94–95
Diplococcus pneumoniae: causing bacterial meningitis, 119
Diplogia, 56
Down's syndrome
 discussion of, 74
 mental retardation in, 59
DPH: in seizures, 28–29
"Drop attacks," 23
Dysarthria, 144
Dyscalculia, 137
Dysgraphia, 137
Dyslexia, 137
Dystonia musculorum deformans, 88
Dystrophy
 infantile neuroaxonal, 86
 muscular, 112–114

E

EEG: in seizure disorders, 25–27
Electroencephalography: in seizure disorders, 25–27
Encephalitis, 116
 discussion of, 122
 headache due to, 40
 postinfectious, 122
Encephalocele, 52
Encephalomyelopathy: subacute necrotizing, 86–87
Environmental causes: of mental retardation, 67
Epilepsy
 definition of, 21
 symptomatic, causes of, 21
Epileptic aphasia: acquired, 149
Ergot preparations: in cluster headaches, 37
Ergotamines: in migraines, 35–36
Escherichia coli: causing bacterial meningitis, 118
Ethosuximide: in seizures, 29

F

Febrile seizures, 24–25
  characteristics of, 25
"Fetal Alcohol Syndrome," 66
Fontanelles, 2–3
  in meningitis, 117
Friedreich's ataxia, 89
Fungal meningitis, 121–122

G

Galactosemia, 78–79
Ganglia: basal, degenerative diseases of, 88
Gangliosidoses, 81
Gargoylism, 79–80
Gaucher's disease, 81
Genes, 70–72
Genetic causes: of mental retardation, 59–62
Genetic disorders, 69–84
Gerstmann syndrome, 134, 137
Globoid cell leukodystrophy, 87
Glycogen storage disease: type II, 79
Grand mal seizure, 22–23
Gray matter: degenerative diseases of, 85–87
Guillain-Barré syndrome, 107
Gyrus, 1

H

Hand size: in spastic hemiplegia, 97
Head
  lag, normal, 2
  "tower," 48
  transillumination of, 17
Headaches, 33–41
  classification of, 34
  cluster, 36–37
  depression, 38
  migraine, 33–36
    phases of, 33–34
  post-traumatic, 39
  resulting from underlying neurologic disease, 39–41
  sinus, 38
  tension, 37–38
Hemiatrophy: of brain, 46
Hemiplegia, spastic, 95–97
  hand size in, 97
  posture in, 96
Hemophilus influenzae: causing bacterial meningitis, 118–119
Hemorrhage: intracranial, CT scan in, 56
Holoprosencephaly, 5–6
Homocystinuria, 76–77
Hormone: adrenocorticotropic, in seizures, 30
Horn cell (*see* Anterior horn cell)
Huntington's chorea, 88
Hurler's syndrome, 79–80
Hydrocephalus, 43–45
  CT scan in, 44
  noncommunicating, 43
Hyperactive behavior (*See also* Hyperactivity) causes of, 126–127
Hyperactivity
  constitutional, 126
  definition of, 125
  situational, 126
  syndromes, 125–132
    alternative approaches to therapy, 130–132
    medications in, stimulant, 128–129
    prognosis in, 132
    tranquilizers in, 129–130
    treatment of, 127–130
Hyperglycinemia: ketotic, 78
Hyperventilation: in neurologic examination, 18
Hypoglycemia: causing mental retardation, 64

INDEX

Hyponatremia: causing mental retardation, 64
Hypothyroidism, 82
Hypotonia: definition of, 91

I

Imipramine: in hyperactive behavior, 130
Infancy: massive myoclonic seizures of, 23–24
Infantile
 neuroaxonal dystrophy, 86
 paralysis, 104–105
 spasms, 23–24
Infarction: cerebral, 45
Infections
 central nervous system, 116–124
 congenital, causing mental retardation, 63
Infectious causes: of mental retardation, 63
Intracranial calcifications: in Sturge-Weber syndrome, 61, 62
Intracranial hemorrhage: CT scan in, 56
Isovaleric acidemia, 78

J

Juvenile myasthenia, 111

K

Kernicterus: causing choreoathetosis, 98
Ketotic hyperglycinemia, 78
Klippel-Feil syndrome, 54
Krabbe's disease, 87
Kugelberg-Welander syndrome, 105

L

Language
 development, normal, 141–143
 disorders, 141–150
Lead poisoning: causing mental retardation, 65–66
Learning disabilities, 133–140
 causes of, 134
 definition of, 133
 management of child with, 138–140
 potential, identification of child with, 134–136
 special problems of child with, 140
 types of, 136–137
 underlying problems associated with, 137–138
Leigh's disease, 86–87
Lesch-Nyhan syndrome, 81–82
Leukodystrophy
 globoid cell, 87
 metachromatic, 87
Lipid metabolism: inborn errors of, 81
Lou Gehrig's disease, 105–106
Lumbar vertebra (*see* Vertebra, lumbar)

M

Macewen's sign, 18
Malformations
 Arnold-Chiari, 47–48
 arteriovenous, 54
 cerebellar, 46–48
 cerebral, 42–46
Maple syrup urine disease, 76
Mass lesions: of nervous system, 54–57
Mebaral: in seizures, 28
Megavitamin therapy: in hyperactivity syndromes, 131
Mellaril: in hyperactivity syndromes, 129–130
Meninges, 2
Meningitis, 116–122
 aseptic, 120–121

Meningitis *(cont.)*
  bacterial, 117–120
    types of, 118
  fungal, 121–122
  headache due to, 40
  tuberculous, 120
  viral, 120–121
Meningocele, 50, 51
Meningoencephalitis, 116
Meningomyelocele, 50–52
Menkes' kinky hair syndrome, 86
Mental retardation, 58–68
  care of child with, 67–68
  causes of, 59–67
  congenital causes of, 62–63
  environmental causes of, 67
  genetic causes of, 59–62
  hyperactive behavior and, 126–127
  infections causing, congenital, 63
  infectious causes of, 63
  metabolic causes of, 63–65
  toxins causing, 65–66
  trauma causing, 66–67
Mental status: evaluation of, 13
Mephobarbital: in seizures, 28
Metabolic causes: of mental retardation, 63–65
Metabolic disorders, 69–84
Metachromatic leukodystrophy, 87
Methylphenidate: in hyperactivity syndromes, 128–129
Methysergide in headaches
  cluster, 37
  migraine, 36
Microcephaly, 3, 45
Microgyria, 43
Migraine, 33–36
  phases of, 33–34
Mongolism (*see* Down's syndrome)
Moro reflex, 4–5
Motor seizures, 24

Motor skills: evaluation of, 16
Motor unit, 103
  schematic representation of, 103
MSUD, 76
Mucopolysaccharidoses, 79–80
  classification of, 80
Muscle
  atrophy
    peroneal, 89
    spinal, 105
  diseases, 103–115
  dystrophy, 112–114
  tone, evaluation of, 14
Myasthenia gravis, 109–112
  congenital, 110–111
  juvenile, 111
  transient neonatal, 110
Myelin, 106
Myoclonic seizures: of infancy, massive, 23–24
Myoclonus: segmental, 24
Myopathy, 104
  acquired, 114
  congenital, 114
Mysoline: in seizures, 29

N

Neck
  reflex, tonic, 4
  stiff, in meningitis, 117
Neimann-Pick disease, 81
Neisseria meningitidis: causing bacterial meningitis, 119
Neonatal myasthenia: transient, 110
Nerve(s)
  cranial, evaluation of, 13, 14
  diseases, 103–115
  peripheral, disorders of, 106–108
Nervous system
  autonomic, evaluation of, 16
  central, infections of, 116–124

INDEX

degenerative diseases of, 85–89
mass lesions of, 54–57
structural diseases of, 42–57
tumors of, 55
Neuroaxonal dystrophy: infantile, 86
Neurocutaneous syndromes, 72
mental retardation and, 59
Neurofibromatosis, 72–74
Neurologic development
milestones
birth to 6 months, 6–8
early school years, 10–11
second year of life, 9
six to twelve months, 8
third to fifth year, 9–10
normal, 1–11
birth to 6 months, 3–6
skills acquired during first year of life, 5
Neurologic disease: causing headache, 39–41
Neurologic examination, 12–20
Neuromuscular junction, 104
diseases of, 108–112
Neuropathy, 104
peripheral, 106
Nevus: port-wine, in Sturge-Weber syndrome, 60

O

Organic acids: disorders of, 78
Orthopedic devices: in cerebral palsy, 99–101
Oxycephaly, 48

P

Palsy
bulbar, 112
cerebral (*see* Cerebral palsy)
pseudobulbar, 94
Panencephalitis: subacute sclerosing, 86
Papilledema, 56
Paralysis: infantile, 104–105
Paresis: definition of, 91
Pemoline: in hyperactivity syndromes, 129
Peroneal muscular atrophy, 89
Petit mal seizure, 23
Phenobarbital
in hyperactive behavior, 126–127
in seizures, 28
Phenylketonuria
discussion of, 75–76
mental retardation in, 62
Photophobia: in meningitis, 117
PKU (*see* Phenylketonuria)
Placing reflex, 5–6
Plagiocephaly, 48
Plegia: definition of, 91
Poisoning: lead, causing mental retardation, 65–66
Poliodystrophy: progressive, 85–86
Poliomyelitis, 104–105
Polyneuritis: postinfectious, 107
Pompe's disease, 79
Porencephaly, 45–46
CT scan in, 46
Port-wine nevus: in Sturge-Weber syndrome, 60
Postinfectious encephalitis, 122
Postinfectious polyneuritis, 107
Post-traumatic headaches, 39
Posture
in spastic hemiplegia, 96
in spastic quadriplegia, 93
Primidone: in seizures, 29
Propionic acidemia, 78
Pseudobulbar palsy, 94
Pseudobulbar speech, 144–145
Pseudotumor cerebri: causing headache, 40
Psychomotor seizures, 23

Q

Quadriplegia, spastic, 93–94
chair for infant with, 101
posture in, 93

R

Reflex(es)
  deep tendon, testing of, 13–14
  developmental, testing of, 16–17
  Moro, 4–5
  placing, 5–6
  stepping, 5–6
  tonic neck, 4
Rehabilitative therapy: in cerebral palsy, 99
Retardation (*see* Mental retardation)
Reye's syndrome: causing mental retardation, 65
Ritalin: in hyperactivity syndromes, 128–129

S

Sacral agenesis, 52–54
Scan (*see* CT scan)
Scaphocephaly, 48
Sclerosis
  amyotrophic lateral, 105–106
  tuberous, 59–60
Segmental myoclonus, 24
Seizure(s)
  adversive, 24
  akinetic, 23
  disorders, 21–32
    headache due to, 40–41
    prognosis, 31
    treatment of, 27–31
  febrile, 24–25
    characteristics of, 25
  focal, 24
  generalized, 22–24
  grand mal, 22–23
  of infancy, massive myoclonic, 23–24
  management of, 32
  motor, 24
  petit mal, 23
  psychomotor, 23
  recurrent, precautions for children with, 31–32
  sensory, 24
  types of, 22
Sensation: examination of, 15–16
Sensory seizures, 24
Sex-linked traits, 70
Sinus headaches, 38
Skills
  auditory retention, 147
  design copying, age acheived at, 10
  during first year of life, 5
  motor, evaluation of, 16
Sodium valproate: in seizures, 30
Spasms: infantile, 23–24
Spastic diplegia, 94–95
Spastic hemiplegia (*see* Hemiplegia, spastic)
Spastic quadriplegia (*see* Quadriplegia, spastic)
Spasticity: definition of, 91
Speech
  ataxic, 145
  creative, 142
  development, normal, 141–143
  disorders, 141–150
  production, disorders of, 143–146
  pseudobulbar, 144–145
Spina bifida, 49–52
  occulta, 49
Spinal cord anomalies, 49–54
Spinal muscular atrophies, 105
Spinocerebellar degenerations, 89
SSPE, 86
Staphylococcus aureus: causing bacterial meningitis, 117–118
Stenosis: aqueductal, 43
Stepping reflex, 5–6

INDEX 161

Stimulants: in hyperactivity syndromes, 128–129
Structural diseases: of nervous system, 42–57
Sturge-Weber syndrome, 61–62
  intracranial calcifications in, 61, 62
  port-wine nevus in, 60
Stuttering, 145–146
Sulcus, 1
Surgery: in cerebral palsy, 101
Sutures, 2
Syringomyelia, 53–54

T

Tay-Sachs disease, 72, 81
Tegretol: in seizures, 29–30
Tendon reflexes: deep, testing of, 13–14
Tension headaches, 37–38
Thioridazine: in hyperactivity syndromes, 129–130
Thorazine: in hyperactivity syndromes, 130
Tofranil: in hyperactivity syndromes, 130
Tomography (see CT scan)
Tonic neck reflex, 4
"Tower head," 48
Toxins: causing mental retardation, 65–66
Traction response, 17
Traits
  autosomal, 70
  sex-linked, 70
Tranquilizers: in hyperactivity syndromes, 129–130
Transillumination: of head, 17
Trauma
  headaches after, 39
  mental retardation due to, 66–67
Trichopoliodystrophy, 86
Tuberculous meningitis, 120
Tuberous sclerosis, 59–60
Tumors
  brain (see Brain, tumors)
  nervous system, 55

U

Urea cycle defects, 77–78

V

Valium: in cerebral palsy, 98–99
Variable penetrance, 71
Ventricles, 2
Vertebra
  defects, 49–54
  lumbar
    bifid defect in, 50
    diagram of, 49
Viral meningitis, 120–121

W

Werdnig-Hoffmann disease, 105
White matter: degenerative diseases of, 87
Wilson's disease, 88

Z

Zarontin: in seizures, 29